EPIDEMIOLOGICAL, DIAGNOSTIC AND THERAPEUTIC SPECIFICITIES OF GYNAECOLOGICAL, BREAST AND UROLOGICAL CANCERS IN CAMEROON

Under the supervision of

Professor Jean YOMI

EPIDEMIOLOGICAL, DIAGNOSTIC AND THERAPEUTIC SPECIFICITIES OF GYNAECOLOGICAL, BREAST AND UROLOGICAL CANCERS IN CAMEROON

Preface by Mama Fouda André

L'Harmattan

By the same author

Particularités épidémiologiques et thérapeutiques des cancers gynécologiques et urologiques au Cameroun, 2018.

5-7, rue de l'École-Polytechnique, 75005 Paris
http://www.editions-harmattan.fr
ISBN : 978-2-343-15915-7
EAN : 9782343159157

CONTRIBUTIONS

Blaise NKEGOUM

University Professor and Hospital Practitioner
Professor of Anatomopathology
Anatomopathology Department
University Teaching Hospital, Yaounde

Etienne ATENGUENA

Medical Doctor, Medical oncologist
Medical Oncology Department
Yaounde General Hospital

Roméo TALLA FOGANG

Master in Radiology and Medical imaging
PhD student in Medical Radiophysics
Centre of Atomic and Molecular Physics
And Quantum Optics (CEPAMOQ), Douala University

Armel DOUANLA BOGNING

Master in Radiology and Medical Imaging
Higher Institute of Applied Technology
And Management (ISTAG), Yaounde

Aristide Donald NGUENDJIO YOMI

Engineer in Statistics and Economics
National Institute of Statistics, Yaounde

PREFACE

According to WHO statistics, almost 8.5 million new cases of cancers appear each year in the world, among which the two-thirds will probably involve developing countries like ours, if nothing is done to reverse this trend!

Indeed, in Cameroon, epidemiological data are quite worrying with an incidence rate of 14,000 new cases of cancers and a prevalence of at least 25,000 cases a year. On the basis of these data, cancer would represent the second cause of mortality, morbidity and therefore, the destruction of the economic fabric in our country.

In a such particular alarming context, on high instruction of His Excellency Mr. President of the Republic, a strategic document on the Health sector was produced in 2001, including a National Programme for Fight against Cancer that was validated and implemented in 2003.

In addition to the preventive aspects, the curative part of this Programme takes into account the improvement of cancer care, the training of suitable human resources and the strengthening of current infrastructures in the two Radiotherapy Departments created in 1987 in the General hospitals of Yaounde and Douala.

We warmly thank the authors of this very first handbook of cancerology whose both versions, French and English, would certainly be in an asset with the promotion of bilingualism and multiculturalism advocated by the Head of State. This work will bring to every Cameroonian or patient, general practitioners and specialists, paramedical staff and NGOs, specific oncological information of an epidemiological, preventive, diagnostic and therapeutic aspects, which are essential for a victorious holistic fight against cancer in Cameroon.

The Minister of Public Health of Cameroon

MAMA FOUDA André

FOREWORD

Contrary to the initial absolutely casuistry conception, nowadays, cancer is not at all known as an exclusive disease of " white " men; it is also and especially the disease of " black " men, mostly in developing countries.

Indeed, according to WHO statistics, 8.5 million new cases of cancers appear each year in the world, among which the two-thirds would probably involve developing countries like Cameroon, if the measures taken to fight against this disease are not sufficiently effective to reverse this trend.

Nowadays, experts unanimously recognise that the non-existence of qualified human resources, the ignorance of the populations and especially the great seriousness of nutritional, parasitic and infectious pandemics over the years of independence have constituted the main causes which have for a long time, created a diversion and forced to limit the general objective of the pseudo-first stage of the fight against cancers in low-income countries, to its non-scientific existence.

The second stage of the fight, then well justified by the demonstration of the existence of cancer pathology in Africans, will effectively begin after the scientific Days of Dakar in 1963 with the communications of SANKALE and the publications of R. ESSOMBA, ANOMAH NGU and ZOUNG KANYI in the 1970s.

Unfortunately, this second stage well initiated and that began so well, will quickly be crystallised around socio-economic, technological, educational and even organisational obstacles, whose major consequence is the inequality of access to health care, resulting in the increase of many cancer care areas administratively and scientifically not approved. Such an organisation could only lead to a heterogeneous, ineffective and dangerous proliferation of various types of treatment protocols, whose implementation strategies are rather individual and competitive than multidisciplinary and concerted. These strategies are therefore the cause of many omissions, mistakes, diagnostic delays and especially therapeutic faults.

This very first handbook of clinical cancerology in Cameroon in both French and English versions would like to be considered within the framework of bilingualism and multiculturalism in force in our country. It is a training tool which could not play the role of a concise handbook considering the extreme complexity and the magnitude of the topic. It should neither be considered as an exhaustive treatise, already available in our university libraries. It is simply a didactic book, whose content based on over 30 years experience in oncologic practice aims to put at the disposal of each Cameroonian without any exception, epidemiological, diagnostic, therapeutic and preventive specificities of cancers found in Cameroon. That will enable them to understand and contribute to the effective implementation of a comprehensive policy of the fight against cancers in our country.

Concretely, the ultimate goal is to bring the whole population, the patients in particular, medical students, general practitioners, medical specialists, paramedical staff and NGOs, to contribute to the setting up of optimum conditions, suitable for curative and early preventive care, through protocol standardisation and organisation that will enable a significant improvement of the quality of care and a visible reduction of mortality and morbidity, due to cancer in our country.

After this first volume on gynaecological and urological cancers, we are willing to gradually write volumes relating to other systems.

The Author

Pr Jean YOMI

PART ONE

GYNAECOLOGICAL AND BREAST CANCERS

Breast cancers

I. Epidemiological specificities

It is the first female cancer in Cameroon and in developed countries. It is proved that one woman over ten will be affected by this cancer during her life.

Its incidence is at least one million new cases per year worldwide. According to the statistics of the National Committee for the Fight against Cancers in Cameroon (CNLC), it represents 21.5% of all cancers and 4 to 6% occur in men.

The age at diagnosis in developed countries is around 50-54; it is even lower in Cameroon with an average age of 40.

The risk factors are represented by:

– Age : the frequency increases with the age

– Sex : more frequent in women than in men (4 to 6%).

– Hormonal Factors mainly related to a long period of oestrogenic impregnation:

- Age more than 30 at the first pregnancy
- Age at early puberty lower than 13 and age more than 55 at late menopause.

– Benign diseases of the breast

- Fibrocystic disease associated with proliferative hyperplasia

– Family and genetic Factors

- Family medical history of breast cancer

- Altered forms of tumour suppressor genes: P53, BRCA1, and BRCA2

– Ionising Radiations

– Viruses

II. Diagnostic procedure

Breast cancer is often suspected on the basis of several symptoms, such as:

- Breast pain
- Unilateral and single canal nipple discharge of lactescent, clear or bloody aspect
- Breast distortion in the form of a nipple retraction, orange peel or thickness
- Presence of lump or lymph nodes after self-fortuitous palpation of breast or axillary crease
- The diagnosis is directed by the following clinical signs:
- Breast distortion in the form of a nipple retraction, orange peel or thickness
- Breast nodule
- Cervico sus-clavicular and axillary lymph nodes

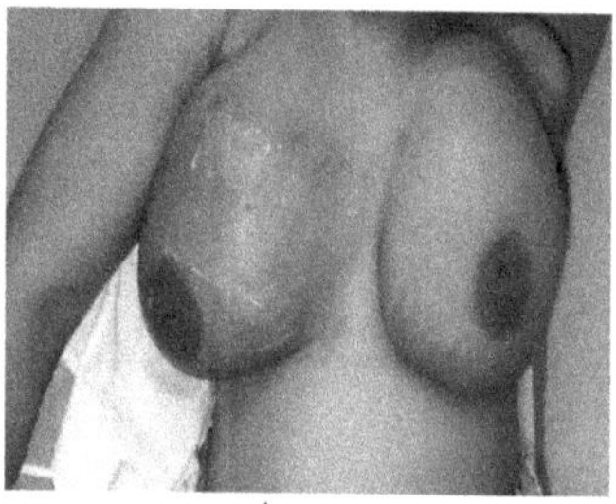

A

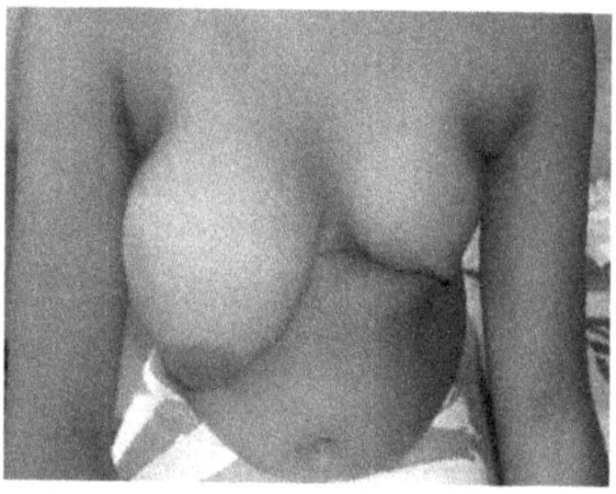

B

Breast Burkitt Lymphoma

A : Bilateral form in a pregnant woman of 20 years old

B : right Breast Unilateral form in a teenager of 16 years old

This diagnosis is confirmed on the base of the Couple echography/mammography results:

- Breast nodules,
- Crervico sus-clavicular and axillary lymph nodes,
- Micro calcifications

The diagnosis is confirmed on the base of histological proof after anatomopathological study of the biopsy punch or the micro-biopsy product by drill or trut cut. However, for economic reasons, in our daily practice, we often accepted the results of cytology after needle tumour aspiration in spite of their relative values particularly operator dependent.

Anatomopathology results

They should be given in the form of a standardised report according to the following model.

STANDARD EXAMPLE OF ANATOMOPATHOLOGICAL EXAM REPORT

1. Identification of the patient :
   - Surname, Given name, sex, age,
   - Residence area,
   - Personal and family medical history of tumour
2. Accessible anatomo-clinical data in Cameroon
   - TNM stage pathological data:
   - Histological description
     - histologic types
     - In-situ contingent
     - Histoprognostic grade
     - State of surgical margins after conservative treatment
     - Presence of peripheral tumour vascular embols
     - Neural infiltration

- Uni or multifocal lesions
- Number of positive nodes under the total nodes removed
- PTNM stage

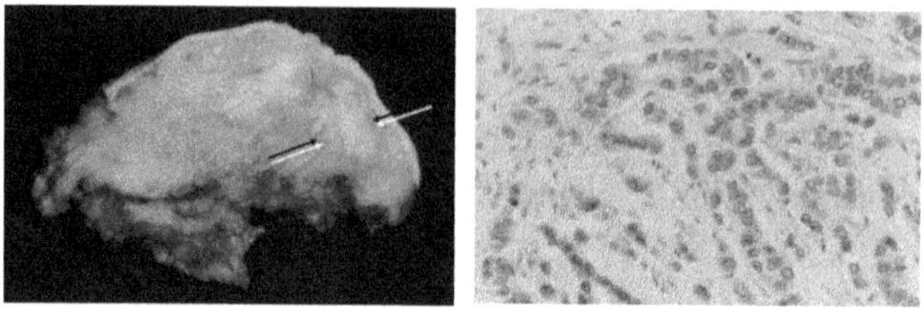

A **B**

Breast carcinoma

A : Macroscopic specimen

B : Histology (Hemateine-eosine technique)

3. Anatomo-clinical data not yet spontaneously accessible in Cameroon

- Hormonal receptor expression level (OR and PR), Ki67
- HER2 receptor expression level
- Molecular genetics (FISH, Oncotype DX and others)
- Molecular sub-types: luminal A, luminal B, HER2 and Triple negative Status

More than the two main histologic types often met in literature, adenocarcinomas and sarcoma in 98% and 2% of cases respectively, Burkitt's lymphomas particularly, are not so rare among relatively young patients in our series.

III. Assessment of tumoral extension and the patient

- ***Assessment of tumoral extension***

- Locally, it aims at specifying the primitive site of the tumour and to estimate its size or volume by means of breast clinical palpation and medical imaging using echography-mammography couple.

- The evaluation of regional extension at the levels of nodal areas of internal mammary, axillary and cervico-sus-clavicular chains will be done by the palpation of clinically accessible areas and medical imaging using echography, CT-scan or lympho scintigraphy although unavailable in our hospital milieu, indicated for deep node chains and sentinel lymph node research.

- The evaluation of remote extension or metastases will be done with the help of symptomatology guided medical imaging for economic reasons at the pleuropulmonal, hepatic, bone and central nervous system levels. Therefore, standard radiography and echography have been very often used; CT-scan, bone scintigraphy, especially MRI, have been sometimes prescribed, but rarely systematically performed due to long time breakdowns of the machines or to high costs of these exams. It is relevant to highlight the importance of fusing imaging techniques (PET/SCAN) and Ca 15-3 more specific tumour marker measurement. Unfortunately, all these high-tech imaging and biological equipments are not yet spontaneously available.

- ***Pre-therapeutic assessment of the patient***

Its aim is to evaluate the patient general status and to detect defects as cardio-respiratory, renal, liver insufficiency, biological and immunological abnormalities. For this purpose, clinical, radiological and biological means have been very often used.

IV. Classification and prognostic factors

- ***Classification :*** *TNM*

Tis : In-situ carcinoma

T1: ≤ 2 cm

T2: ≥ 2 cm and ≤ 5 cm in its greater dimension

T3: $\geq$ 5 cm in its greater dimension

T4: tumour of any size with direct extension to the thoracic wall or to the skin.

- T4a: Extension to the thoracic wall
- T4b: oedema or skin ulceration or cutaneous nodules confined in the same breast;
- T4c: T4a + b
- T4d: inflammatory breast (PEV 2 and 3);

N1: Homolateral axillary mobile lymphadenopathies;

N2: Homolateral axillary fixed lymphadenopathies;

N3: Lymphadenopathies of the homolateral internal mammary chain;

M1: Remote metastases, including sus-clavicular lymphadenopathies.

Prognostic factors and degrees of severity:

Degree of severity / **Prognostic factors**	*Good prognosis*	*Poor prognosis*
TNM Stage	T_0, T_1, T_2< 3 cm N_0 et N≤ 3cm M_0	T2, T3 > 3 cm ; T4 N> 3 cm M_1
SBR Grade	SBR I and SBR II	SBR III
Rh : Oestrogen, Progesterone	Rh^+ POSITIVE	Rh^- NEGATIVE
HER 2	HER 2^+ POSITIVE	HER 2^- NEGATIVE
Triple negative status	Absent	Present
Clinical status of the patient	Good general status	Bad general status

V. Therapeutic methods

Three therapeutic methods are frequently used, rarely exclusively but very often in association:

- *The surgery*

It is a loco-regional means of treatment which is applied according to two radical and conservative methods: total mastectomy associated with homolateral axillary dissection according to PATEY, and lumpectomy or quadrantectomy; corresponding to radical and conservative surgery respectively.

The indications of conservative surgery are mainly: single site primary tumour with a size $\leq$ 3 cm and a suitable breast volume, then, larger size tumours at T_2, T_3 stages or multiple site tumours are the main indications for radical surgery technique.

Lobular carcinoma or intra-canal histology type and phyllode tumours, not forgetting the inaccessibility to a radiotherapy treatment, represent the main contraindications for conservative surgery.

- *The radiotherapy*

As surgery, it is a loco regional method of breast cancer treatment using ionising radiations (X and ɣ rays).

The radiotherapy planning is an essential step with the objective to determine the main irradiation parameters:

> **Patient position on the treatment machine**

The supine position on an inclined plan, particularly comfortable, easy to perform, maintain and especially to reproduce has always been adopted.

> **Target Volumes**

The three main target volumes that will be irradiated must be delimited and simulated with precision

- V1 = Breast + thoracic wall in case of conservative treatment
- V2 = Thoracic wall + mastectomy scar in case of radical treatment
- V3 = Axillo sus-clavicular and CMI lymph nodes

➢ **Total dose of the treatment**

It ranges from 45 to 50 Gy with a possible tumoral bed boost of 10 to 15 Gy

➢ **Nature of the radiation used**

The co60 gamma ray of 1. 25 MeV or the X-ray of 10-15 MeV of the linear accelerator can be used, according to equipment possibilities.

➢ **Fractionation**

Classically, 05 fractions of 2 Gy are delivered a week at the rate of one fraction a day.

➢ **Spreading**

This parameter is defined as the total duration of the treatment which ranges from 4 to 5 weeks for a total dose of 45-50 Gy.

➢ **Organs at risk to be protected**

With personalised and well placed blocks, we should protect organs at risk such as: larynx, deltoid muscle, lungs, clavicle, heart, cervico-thoracic spinal cord.

➢ **Proper technical Preparation of the irradiation**

It is done in three main phases of equal importance:

- Simulation : its objective is to determine with the use of a simulator, all necessary geometrical and mechanical parameters of the irradiation of target volumes.

- The computer-assisted dosimetry enables estimating pre-treatment distribution of doses in the target volumes and organs at risk. It also allows the necessary modifications and permits the radiation oncologist to validate the final dosimetry plan.
- After the patient's installation on the treatment machine, the radiation treatment can start.

▪ ***The chemotherapy***

It is the main loco-regional and systemic means of treatment. Nowadays, it is done with a poly chemotherapy protocol. The targeted therapy, unfortunately much less used due to its high cost, is, however, recommended for positive HER2 receptor tumours.

▪ ***The hormonotherapy***

Its action which is also local, regional and systemic is only useful in case of positivity of oestrogen and progesterone hormonal receptors.

Two methods of administration are generally used:

- Subtractive by means of a surgical castration, through a bilateral ovariectomy or radiotherapy delivering a total dose of 12 Gy in 3 fractions in 3 days in the mean frontal plan of pelvis.
- Additive by a parenteral administration of LH-RH agonists or oral administration of Tamoxifen at the dose of 20 mg a day for 5 years. This method known as chemical castration has replaced the subtractive method which is no more practically used.

VI. Indications and therapeutic protocols

Indications	Therapeutic protocols
$T_1T_2 \leq 3$ cm (single, normal site, normal breast volume)	Conservative treatment : ➢ Surgery: lumpectomy + axillary dissection ➢ Radiotherapy: 45 Gy-50 Gy (10-15 Gy)
BIG T_2, T_3, T_{4a}	Radical treatment ➢ Surgery: mastectomy + axillary dissection ➢ Radiotherapy: 45 Gy /22f /4-5 weeks
T_1 T_2, T_3, T_{4a} N^+ RH^+ SBRII + III **Pre-menopausal women**	➢ Polychemotherapy + subtractive hormonotherapy + surgery + radiotherapy
T_1 T_2, T_3, T_{4a} N^+ RH^+ SBRII + III **Menopausal women**	Age>70 : ➢ RH^+ additive hormonotherapy Age<70 (poor prognostic factors RH^- SBR III) : ➢ Hormonotherapy + Poly-chemotherapy + surgery + radiotherapy
$T_{4b}T_{4c}$ inflammatory:	➢ Poly chemotherapy + surgery + radiotherapy + hormonotherapy
T_{4d} metastasis:	➢ Poly chemotherapy ± cleaning surgery ± radiotherapy with a palliative goal of bone/cerebral metastasis (30 Gy/10 F/12D or 20 Gy/5 F/4D)

VII. current therapeutic Results, means and fellow-up methods

- ***Current results***

The results are significantly good for early stages with good prognosis, unfortunately very rare in our hospitals.

- **T 1, T 2:**
  - Survival rate (SR) in 10 years : 75-80 %
  - Local recurrence rate: 4-10%
- **T 3, T 4:**
  - Overall SR: in 5 years : 45-50 %

- ***Follow-up***

During the treatment, our attention should be focused on the research of dysphasia or epithelitis on the preserved breast or thoracic wall in case of a mastectomy, axillary and cervico-sus-clavicular fossa. Usually, these lesions are easily treated with simple medical care.

In the long term, breast oedema, top pulmonary fibrosis, swollen arms and shoulders join ankylosis are the main handicaps feared, difficult to treat by physiotherapy and lymphatic drainage.

Long term planning of such a follow-up should take into account the clinical status of the patient. In general, it will be quarterly the first year, semi-annual the second year, then yearly from the 3rd year, up to 5 years at least.

Clinical exams, chest X-ray, annual mammography with reduced incidence number and breast echography, will be the main follow-up means. The prescription of other examination methods such as bone scintigraphy, CT Scan and MRI should be for economic reasons guided by symptomatology.

VIII. Essential preventive Measures and prospects

- Healthy and balanced diet and physical exercise are the main recommended primary preventive measures.
- Mammography screening and the search for genetic advice for family high-risk patients are the main measures of secondary prevention which must be initiated and developed in specialised centres.
- The improvement of the current results will only be possible if socio-economic measures are improved, enabling the accessibility to new therapies, in particular, the targeted ones, taking into account the tumour genomics data for triple negative status.

Cervical cancers

I. Epidemiological specificities

Cervical cancer is known to be very frequent in developing countries such as Cameroon. It ranks second after breast cancers in women.

According to Globocan 2012 data, updated and validated by the national committee for fight against cancers in Cameroon, its incidence is estimated at 20/100,000 a year with a mortality rate of 3.1 deaths/ 100,000 women.

Clinically, the average age at the diagnosis is 55 or 60 in the West, it is even lower (35 or 40) in developing countries.

Etiological factors for which cause-and-effect relationship was demonstrated are mainly represented by infections namely, HPV (Human Papilloma Virus), HIV especially, and smoking. Poverty, obstetrical trauma due to the high multiparty, obstetrical instrumentations, multiple sexual partners, are just favouring factors.

II. Diagnostic procedure

The diagnosis is essentially late in developing countries. Indeed, at least 80% of patients are seen at late stages, most often due to economic reasons and the long distance to specialised hospitals, but unfortunately, because of ignorance, the negative role played by traditional healers, ''therapeutic'' prayer houses and other taboos.

However, it is known to be a pathology with a very rich and early symptomatology. Vaginal bleeding is very frequent and can be pre or post menopausal, spontaneous or induced, in particular after sexual intercourse or aggressive genital hygiene. The bleeding may be abundant, requiring the protection by a great quantity of sanitary towels; it may also be in a very limited quantity in the form of a too small stain on the panties that need a special attention of the patient to be discovered.

Purulent and foul-smelling leucorrhoea may coexist with the bleeding, preceding or succeeding it.

The late symptoms corresponding to a quite advanced stage of the disease are mainly constituted by lombo-pelvic pains; signs of bladder and rectal infiltration respectively as pollakiuria, dysuria, then, false needs and even constipation.

The frequency of asymptomatic forms, usually maintained by carelessness, may be significant, depending on socio-economic and educational living standard of populations. In this context, the essential role of Pap smear screening technique with systematic gynaecological examinations, that can be done individually or during preventive mass campaigns, is not to be demonstrated any more.

Clinically, the gynaecological examination using speculum can enable observing, at the cervix, a lesion in the form of a simple red zone, or irregular shape ulceration with a necrotic background or a variable-sized, friable and haemorrhagic bud. It should be noted that, the cervix may present a pseudo-normal aspect particularly with infra-clinical forms for which a colposcopy guided biopsy following Schiller's test is indicated.

In gynaecological position, the bladder and rectum being emptied, respectively by the installation of a permanent bladder catheter and the rectal enema, the digital pelvic examination (vaginal and rectal) aim at specifying the site, the size, the extension in the parameters, the vesico-vaginal and recto-vaginal septa of the primary tumour.

The general examination of the patient through simple palpation must enable to search for inguino-crural and cervico-sus-clavicular adenopathies to estimate the size and the consistency of the liver.

After being guided by the signs and symptoms described, only the histologic study of the biopsy sample or the Pap smear cytology can permit to confirm the final diagnosis. More often, epidermoid carcinoma and adenocarcinoma, then, sometimes lymphoma and sarcoma are the main histologic types met in 90 and 10% of cases respectively.

III. Assessment of tumoral extension and the patient

- *Assessment of tumoral extension*

Locally, it aims at estimating the site and volume of the primary tumour during gynaecological examination, under general anaesthesia. In addition to digital pelvic examinations already described, the evaluation of the bladder or rectal invasion should be done by cystoscopy and rectoscopy.

Regionally, the invasion of pelvic lymph nodes and surrounding organs will mainly be searched for with morphological examinations such as: echography, Intravenous Urography and sometimes CT Scan in spite of their limited value. The functional medical imaging such as MRI (Magnetic Resonance Imaging) or even better, 18-FDG PET-SCAN image fusion is optional for its effectiveness, but unfortunately very expensive, therefore, less accessible in our hospitals.

The distant extension will be assessed by means echography, Standard Radiography, CT Scan and/or MRI and bone scintigraphy according to cases. For economic and effectiveness reasons, the prescription of all these examinations should be guided as far as possible by symptomatological and clinical data.

- ***Patient status evaluation***

Its aim is to evaluate the general status of the patient and to search for defects which can be from haematological, cardiopulmonary, diabetic, renal, hepatic and immunological origin, by using well indicated clinical, radiological and biological tests.

IV. Classification and prognostic factors

This classification is that of the International Federation of Gynaecologists and Obstetricians (FIGO), mainly based on clinical and paraclinical data.

- FIGO staging

FIGO stages	Description
I	**Carcinoma confined to the cervix**
IA	Invasive carcinoma diagnosed only by microscopy
IA1	Micro invasive carcinoma < 3 mm in depth and < 7 mm stromal invasion
IA2	Micro invasive carcinoma > 3 mm and < 5 mm in depth and < 7 mm stromal invasion
IB	Clinically visible lesion confined to the cervix or microscopy lesion > IA2
IB1	Lesion < 4 cm
IB2	Lesion > 4 cm
II	**Cervical carcinoma invades beyond uterus but not to the pelvic wall or to the lower-third of the vagina**
IIA	No clinical parametrial invasion
IIB	Clinical extension to the parameters
III	**Clinical extension to the pelvic wall and/or to the lower-third of the vagina. Any case with hydronephrosis or non-functional kidney corresponds to stage III**
IIIA	Extension to the lower-third of the vagina wall
IIIB	Extension to the parameters until the pelvic wall
IV	**Extension to the bladder or rectum or outside of the pelvis**
IVA	Clinical extension to the bladder or rectum mucosa
IVB	Metastatic extension beyond the pelvis

The main poor prognosis factors are represented by:

- Advanced FIGO stages: III and IV
- Haemoglobin level $\leq$ 12 g/100 ml
- Young age $\leq$ 35 years old
- Poor clinical status of the patient:
    - Performance Status (PS) > 2
    - Karnofsky < 60%

V. Therapeutic methods

- ***The radiation therapy***

Its curative aim is to eradicate the disease at the loco regional stage. Unfortunately, this indication is only possible for less than 20% of our patients received at early FIGO stages, I and IIA.

Its palliative aim is only to improve the general comfort of the patient through its effectiveness on pain relieve, haemostatic action, pelvic, bone and cerebral decompression, in more than 80% of the cases late diagnosed and treated in our hospitals.

Radiation therapy techniques

Two main techniques are often used:

- External Radiation therapy or tele radiation therapy: defined as such, because the radioactive source is placed outside and at a certain distance from the patient.

The irradiation parameters to be determined with a simulator by the radiation oncologist are mainly :

i- The patient position on the treatment machine : the supine position, easily carried out and reproducible is very often adopted

ii- The target volume to be treated, generally the entire pelvis comprising the primary tumour and pelvic lymph nodes;

iii- The curative and palliative total dose, ranges from 45-50 Gy to 20-30 Gy according to the aim of the treatment.

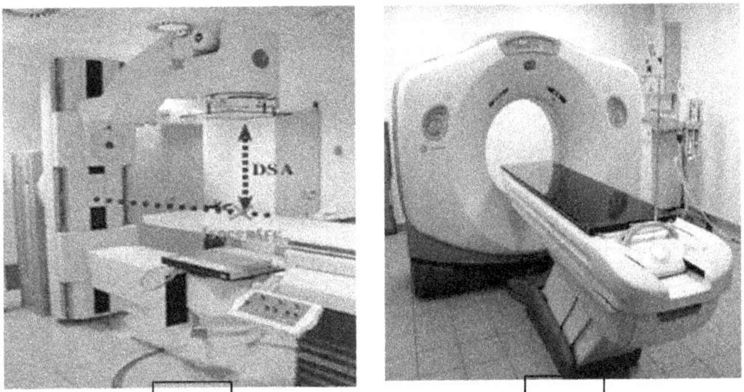

A B

Types of simulator

A : 2D simulator

B : CT-Scan 3D simulator

iv- The planned computer-assisted dosimetry whose role in the improvement of the tolerance and quality of the irradiation is well demonstrated.

- Internal Radiation therapy or Brachytherapy, defined as such, because the radioactive source is rather placed inside the patient. Two sub techniques must be distinguished:
  - If the radioactive source is located near the tumour in a cavity, as the vagina, we will talk about Plesio-Brachytherapy or Endo-Cavitary Brachytherapy.

- Whereas, if the radioactive source is directly inserted in the tumour, we will talk about interstitial brachytherapy or endo-brachytherapy.

With any of these sub brachytherapy techniques, an exclusive total dose of 60-65 Gy or an additional dose of 20-30 Gy after external radiation therapy with 45 Gy may be delivered in a reduced cervico-uterine or vaginal volume.

- ***The surgery***

Its radical curative aim includes a total colpohysterectomy removing the upper one-fourth or one-third of the vagina and a bilateral annexectomy associated with a complete pelvic lymphadenectomy, according to the «Wertheim» or " CHL technique".

In specific cases, it may be partial, conservative, in the form of conisation or supra-vaginal amputation of the cervix with extra pelvic transposition of the ovaries.

- ***The concomitant Association of chemotherapy and radiotherapy***

It is often performed to overcome the radio resistance and especially chemo resistance of some malignant tumours, particularly those of the cervix. For this purpose, Cisplatin and 5-Fluorouracil are the most used molecules for their affordable price, but especially for their radio sensitivity action at low dose.

The main indication of this protocol is: a treatment with a curative aim of relatively young patients, with a good general status, able to tolerate the cumulative toxicity of chemotherapy and radiotherapy.

VI. Indications and therapeutic protocols

Indications	Protocols
Stage 0 – stage IA Young age Pregnancy willingness	➢ CONSERVATIVE SURGERY ➢ Conisation FOLLOW-UP : PAP SMEAR
Stage 0 – stage IA Advanced age and/or adnexal pathology	➢ RADICAL SURGERY ➢ Simple hysterectomy with ovary preservation
Stage IB Young age, T<2 cm	➢ WERTHEIM WITH OVARY TRANSPOSITION
Stage IB Advanced age , T<2 cm	➢ EXTERNAL RADIOTHERAPY + BRACHYTHERAPY
Stage IB – stage II T <2 cm	➢ WERTHEIM, 1st + ovary transposition ➢ Vaginal vault brachytherapy ➢ If N+ : External radiotherapy (ERT)
Stage IB – IIA (proximal) T ≤4 cm	➢ Utero-vaginal brachyttherapy (60 Gy) ➢ Radical surgery: WERTHEIM ➢ N+ : ERT(45 Gy) ➢ N- : FOLLOW-UP
Stage IB – IIA (proximal) T >4 cm	➢ External radiotherapy (45 Gy) ➢ Utero-vaginal brachytherapy (20 Gy) ➢ Radical surgery: WERTHEIM
Stage IB – IIA (proximal) Young age Minor pelvic lymph nodes involvement Minor parameter infiltration No Lombo Aortic lymph nodes involvement.	➢ Concomitant association ERT + chemotherapy
Stage II – III (distal)	➢ ERT (45 Gy) + a boost of 10 G in the parameters ➢ Utero-vaginal brachytherapy (20 Gy)
Stage IV	➢ ERT (45 Gy) + utero-vaginal brachytherapy (20 Gy) or ERT (30 Gy) followed by a posterior or anterior PELVECTOMY

VII. Current therapeutic Results

- ***Current results: 5 years survival rate***
  - **Proximal FIGO I & II :**
    - 80 – 90% if N-
    - 50% if N+
  - **Distal FIGO I &II:**
    - 30 – 40%
  - **FIGO III IV:**
    - Lower than 10%

- ***Follow-up: Aims, Means and Methods***

- During the treatment, medical consultations should be daily organised at the request, with the aim to improve with suitable advice and medical care, the digestive, urinary, cutaneous and vaginal tolerance, which permits the compliance of the patient and the treatment accuracy.
- The follow-up, after the treatment, should be organised in short-and long-term, with the aim to assess the results in terms of complete or partial remission, therapeutic failure, loco regional (centro latero-pelvic) recurrence, by clinical, radiological and biological means. Finally, it will be necessary to search for iatrogenic effects and to facilitate professional, social and family reintegration of the patients.

VIII. Essential preventive measures and prospects

They will have to be institutionalised, organised and implemented during individual consultations and more over during mass campaigns.

- ***Primary preventive measures:***

- Information for the behaviour change
- HPV vaccination for young girls (9 – 13 years old) before the first sexual intercourse or during the year of the first sexual intercourse
- Systematic Treatment for genital infections
- Avoiding active / passive smoking

- ***Secondary preventive measures, using :***

- Screening by one of the usual methods (FCV, VIA/VILI, colposcopy)

- ***Prospects :***

- Generalise the vaccination of the target population
- Institutionalise mass screening campaigns
- Improve access to the best methods and techniques of extension assessment and treatment.

Endometrial cancers

I. Epidemiological specificities

In the West as well as in developing countries, the frequency of endometrial or uterine corpus cancer is constantly growing, with the rise of the economic level; the improvement of life expectancy and the ineffectiveness of primary preventive measures towards etiological factors that are still not well known.

Endometrial cancer, very often occurs around the age of 60. It is observed after 50, in 75% of the cases and only 4% before 40. Sometimes, it will be a post-menopausal, obese, diabetic and hypertensive woman with risks of endogenous or exogenous oestrogen/progesterone imbalance in favour of oestrogen.

However, particularly, in our hospital milieu, more than 40% of endometrial cancers occur without any possibility to establish a cause-effect relation with the hormonal situation.

II. Diagnostic procedure

The most frequent symptom is spontaneous and post-menopausal metrorrhagia. In an age category, the occurrence of metrorrhagia has a relation with a malignant tumour in one-third of the cases. The diagnosis is more difficult to be established during the pre-and-post-menopausal period.

The clinical examination, particularly, the gynaecological type is much less contributory; the cervix and the size of the uterus being generally within the limits of the normal dimensions. Such a lack and very poor signs and symptoms are very often, at the base of the late diagnosis. The groups of high-risk patients at the pre-and-post menopausal age should be explored with the techniques of progressive curettage vacuum extraction of the endometrium under anaesthesia, with an aim to detect pre-cancerous lesions and histologically certifying the diagnosis. For this purpose, the role of hysteroscopy followed by a tumour biopsy is necessary.

In more than 95% of cases, histology is of a well, less and undifferentiated adenocarcinoma type. The myometrium or endometrium sarcoma is met in less than 5% of the cases. Its diagnostic procedure and therapeutic protocols are comparable to those of adenocarcinoma, but particularly individualised by the favourable prognosis of differentiated forms.

III. Assessment of tumoral extension

The tumoral extension at the cervix and proximal parameters level will locally be assessed during the gynaecological examination, leading to specify the seat and estimate the size or the volume of the primary tumour.

Hysteroscopy will be used to evaluate the extension level of the tumour in the uterine cavity and to guide the biopsy.

The regional and distant extension assessment will essentially be done using the medical imaging directed if possible by symptomatology. CT scan and/or abdomino-pelvic MRI will lead to the identification of pelvic and lombo-aortic lymphadenopathies, as well as ovarian tumours, ascites, hepatic and pulmonary involvement.

Assessment of the patient

It is about evaluating the general status of the operability of the patient using clinical, para-clinical and biological examination to detect defects such as: diabetes, high blood pressure, cardio-pulmonary and renal failure.

IV. Anatomopathological and TNM Clinical Classification

It is usually done on the base of macroscopic and microscopic data, from the anatomopathological study of the total tumour after hysterectomy. Its anatomo-clinical aspects and prognostic factors such as: the tumour stage, the degree of differentiation and infiltration of myometrium are the main useful data.

TNM classification

Stages	Description
Stage 0	**Carcinoma in situ**
Stage I	**Tumour confined to the cervix**
IA	Tumour confined to the endometrium
IB	Half thickness of myometrium invasion at most
IC	More than half thickness of myometrium invasion
Stage II	**Tumour cervix extension without exceeding the uterus**
IIA	Invasion confined to endo-cervical glands
IIB	Cervical stroma invasion
Stage III	**Tumour extension out of the uterus**
IIIA	Peritoneum, one annexe or positive peritoneal cytology
IIIB	Continuous or discontinuous vaginal invasion
IIIC	Pelvic and/or lombo-aortic lymph nodes metastases
Stage IV	**Loco-regional organs tumour extension**
IVA	Invasion of vesical and/or rectal mucosa
IVB	Lymph nodes or visceral metastases except the sites described at stage IIIB and IIIC

V. Therapeutic methods and techniques

- *The surgery*

It is the major method of radical treatment of cervical cancers whose technique includes a total hysterectomy, a bilateral annexectomy, iliac and lombo-aortic lymph nodes dissection through a large, supra, para and sub-umbilical median laparotomy.

- *External Radiotherapy*

It may be exclusive in case of non-operability or adjuvant after the surgery.

Parameters of irradiation:

- Position of the patient on the treatment machine: the supine position, easily carried out and reproducible, is most often adopted.
- Target Volume: it is made up of the pelvic cavity and lombo-aortic lymph nodes.
- Total dose : it ranges from 65 Gy to 45-50 Gy depending on the treatment modalities during exclusive or adjuvant radiotherapy.

- *Brachytherapy*

It is usually done using the endo-cavitary brachytherapy technique.

Parameters of irradiation:

- Position of the patient on the treatment machine: supine position as already described.
- Target Volume: vaginal vault after a total hysterectomy or utero-vaginal cavity in case of exclusive brachytherapy when surgery is not indicated.
- Total dose : it ranges from 60 Gy to 20-30 Gy in case of exclusive brachytherapy or after external radiotherapy.

- Aim: prevent any relapses on the vaginal vault after hysterectomy which may occur in 20, to 30 % of the cases.

A

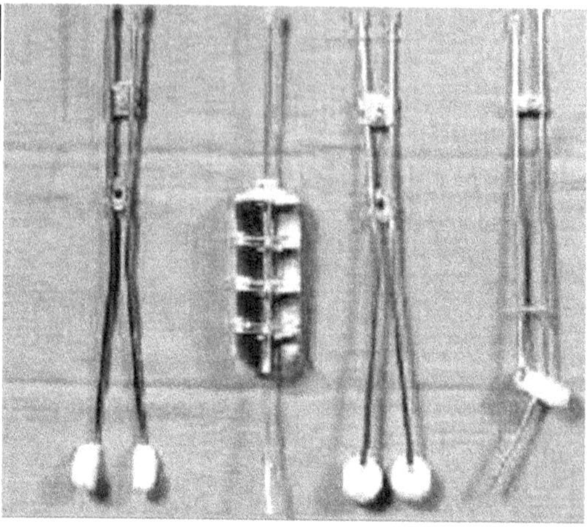

B

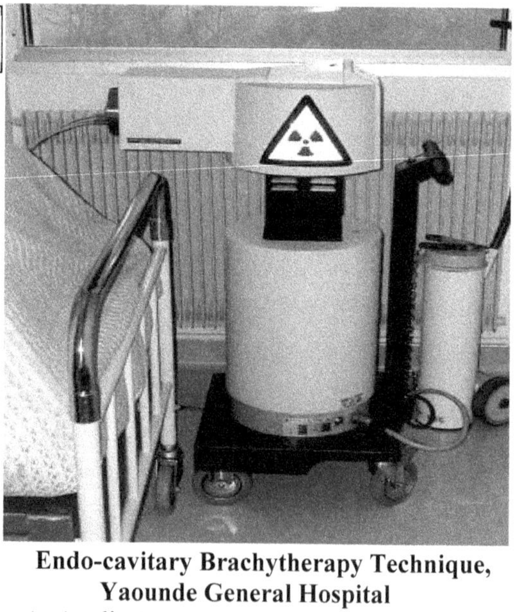

Endo-cavitary Brachytherapy Technique, Yaounde General Hospital

A : Applicators

B : Brachytherapy machine

- ***Hormone therapy***

Additive hormone therapy with progesterone is recommended for advanced stages, metastases cases and recurrence with a low response rate less than 30 %.

- ***Chemotherapy***

It is known to be ineffective on endometrial adenocarcinoma.

VI. Indications and therapeutic protocols

Indications	Therapeutic protocols
Stages I and II - Operable patients - Extirpable tumours - No defect - Well differentiated tumours - Low risk of relapse	Radical surgery + Vaginal vault brachytherapy
Stages I and II Operable patients No defect High risk of recurrence : *cervix ++, *grade III, *myometrium++, *ganglions +++	Radical surgery + External radiotherapy + Vaginal vault brachytherapy
Patients with surgery contraindication	ERT + utero-vaginal brachytherapy
Patients M+ Hormonal receptors+	Hormone therapy AMP :1-3 g/week Tamoxifen : 40 mg/Day Response rate : 30-40%
Patients M+ Hormonal receptors – Hormone therapy failure Tumour degree III	Chemotherapy ADM/CDDP/5 FU/CPM Response rate : 25-30 %

VII. Current results

- Survival Rate (SR): 5 years
- Stage I : 80-85 %
- Degree III: 60%

VIII. Prospects

Develop epidemiological studies in general, and direct them particularly towards the research on the role of endometrial hyperplasia and obesity, then, to guide hormone therapy as far as possible by a systematic study of hormonal receptors.

Gestational and trophoblastic diseases

I. Epidemiological specificities

It is a group of tumours defined as expansive process deriving from trophoblastic tissue. Six entities are distinguished according to the growing degree of malignancy and severity:

- Complete hydatiform mole
- Partial hydatiform mole
- Invasive mole
- Trophoblastic tumour of the placental site
- Tropoblastic tumour of epithelioid type
- Choriocarcinoma

All of them have in common, the production of chorionic gonadotrophic hormone which is the pregnancy hormone.

Its present frequency, estimated at less than 1% of all gynaecological diseases, seems to be under-estimated in the context of the practice in our hospital milieu, where access to anatomopathological examinations of conception products and curettage substances is limited.

The discovery circumstances are all related to the pregnancy:

- Incidence for any type of pregnancy: 1/40,000
- Frequency after molar pregnancy: 1/1,000
- Possible frequency after:
    - Normal pregnancy to term: 1/150,000
    - Ectopic pregnancy
    - Spontaneous or induced abortion

II. Diagnostic procedure

Symptomatology is dominated by an exaggeration of functional signs of pregnancy: nausea, vomiting, breast tension, mainly in a woman with a past medical history of hydatiform mole and miscarriage.

Physical signs are dominated by metrorragia with clinical anaemia complications.

On speculum examination, vaginal secondary tumoral lesions can be discovered.

In addition to the anatomopathological study of curettage substances, the diagnosis of confirmation is necessarily done with the presence of the following FIGO criteria:

- Level of β HCG on 4 values in 4 weeks (D1, D7, D14, D21)
- β HCG over 10% in 3 weeks in 3 values or more (D1, D7, D14)
- High Persistence level of β HCG, 6 months after the evacuation of a molar pregnancy
- Presence of metastases

III. Tumour Extension assessment

The loco regional extension evaluation is to determine the degree of penetration of myometerium, ovary, vagina and other pelvic organs invasion.

The needed methods of evaluation are: the digital clinical pelvic examination and ultrasound, CT Scan or even better MRI of abdominopelvic cavity.

The general status will be assessed by searching for metastases at the level of the most frequent sites which are:

- Lungs (80%)
- Vagina (30%)
- Pelvis (20 %)
- Brain (10%)
- Liver (10%)
- Others (5%)

The most useful methods of evaluation are:

- Clinical examination ;
- Imaging guided by symptomatology;
- However, according to the FIGO recommendations, the chest X-ray is at least recommended in case of pleuropulmonary secondary lesions;
- It will also be necessary to search for occult blood in the stools in case of suspicion of a digestive localisation and to proceed to dosage of β HCG in CSF in case of neuro-meningeal symptomatology with negative imaging of the central nervous system.

Assessment of the patient

It is to assess the general status of the patient and to search for various defects such as diabetes, HTA, renal failure and immunodepression.

Classification (WHO 2000)

Stages	Descriptions
Stage I	Disease confined to the uterus
Stage II	Extension of the disease out of the uterus but confined to genitals (annexes, vagina, broad ligament)
Stage III	Extension to the lungs with or no genitals invasion
Stage IV	Any other metastatic site involvement

IV. Prognostic factors and scores

Scores / Prognoses factors	**0**	**1**	**2**	**4**
Age	≤ 39	> 39		
PMH pregnancy	Mole	Abortion	Birth	
Chemo interval	< 4 months	4 – 6 months	7 – 12 months	> 12 mois
B HCG rate	0 – 1,000	1,000 – 10,000	10,000-100,000	> 100.000
Metastases amount*		1- 4	5 - 8	>8
Metastatic sites		Spleen and kidney	Digestive tract	Brain and silver
Tumour size**		3-5 cm	≥ 5 cm	
Chemo failure			Mono-chemotherapy	Polychimio
Scores <7: low risk of failure to treatment / scores > 7 or stage IV: high risk of failure to treatment				

V. Therapeutic Methods

- *The chemotherapy*

Mono or poly-chemotherapy protocols can be applied, depending on the indications.

> **Mono-chemotherapy protocols:**

- Methotrexate (MTX)
- Actinomycin D (ACT – D)
- Folinic acid (FA)

> **Poly-chemotherapy protocols:**

- (D1) EMA Protocol – CO : Etoposide (VP16) + ACT-D + MTX
- (D2) VP16 protocol + ACT- D + FA
- (D8) Cyclophosphamide (CPM) Protocol + Vincristine (VCR)

- *The surgery*
  - It is a radical surgical method of treatment whose technique includes a total hysterectomy associated with a bilateral annexectomy.
  - In case of hepatic oligometastases, an adjusted hepatectomy may be necessary.

- *The external Radiotherapy*

Its implementation is necessarily done after the determination of several parameters of irradiation by the radiation oncologist:

- Position of the patient on the treatment machine; the supine position is very often adopted for the above-mentioned reasons;
- target Volume: entire pelvis ;

- Total dose : 45 – 50 Gy ;
- Fractionation / total duration of treatment: 5 X 2 Gy a week ;
- The nature of the beam: X-ray of the linear Accelerator with an average energy ranging from 15 to 25 Mev or Gamma-ray of cobalt 60 of 1.25 Mev.

VI. Indications and therapeutic protocols

- Curative aim: To cure the patient and if possible to preserve her fertility

Indications	Therapeutic protocols
Low risk	Mono--chemotherapy (methotrexate)
High risk	Poly-chemotherapy (EMA – CO, BEP)
Unresponsive result	Poly-chemotherapy (EP – EMA)
Uncontrollable haemorrhage	Total hysterectomy + radiotherapy (45-50Gy/5x2Gy/week)
Hepatic metastases	Adjusted hepatectomy

- Palliative aim: To improve the general comfort of the patient

Indications	Therapeutic protocols
Massive uterine haemorrhage	Pelvic radiotherapy (30Gy/10F/12Days) Hysterectomy
Cerebral metastases with intracranial hypertension	Whole-brain radiotherapy (30 Gy/10F / 12 Days)
Hepatic oligometastases	Adjusted hepatectomy + radiotherapy : 20 – 30 Gy (5x3Gy/week)

VII. Current results, Means and Methods of follow-up

- ***Current Results***

The complete response rate and cure is close to 80% on the first line and 75% on the second line of the treatment.

Fertility is almost normal after choriocarcinoma.

- ***Means and Methods of follow-up***

After the treatment, with time, during well-planned consultations, we will carry out clinical, biological and radiological examinations, in order to search for loco regional and remote relapses, not forgetting the abnormalities of subsequent pregnancies which can be authorised only after an optimum time of compulsory contraception.

VIII. Prospects

Only the diagnosis of all cases, possible with the development of a systematic anatomopathological analysis policy of curettage and abortion products, can improve the quality of fight against this pathology, whose negative impact on procreation, is particularly dreaded by patients in general and particularly those in African countries.

Ovarian cancers

I. Epidemiological specificities

In Cameroon, the ovarian malignant tumour represents 3% of all the cancers. It is also the fifth cancer of the Cameroonian woman after the breast, cervical, skin and liver cancer.

The occurrence age is around 60 or more, at least for non-lymphomatous forms.

The risk factor of genetic origin is found in approximately 10 % of the cases. It is often related to BRCA 1 or BRCA 2 genes mutation, and occurs before the age of 60. Unfortunately, the search for such markers still remains technically impossible in our hospital milieu.

The nulliparity, the couple (early menstruation/late menopause) and advanced age are also associated with an increased risk.

The oral contraception, pregnancy, breast feeding and tubal ligation are, however, known as factors of risk reduction of ovarian cancer.

Ovarian cancer is a significant cause of cancer deaths in women, due to its late diagnosis and poor prognosis in 45% of cases in developed countries and at least 70% in low-income countries.

II. Diagnostic procedure

The symptoms and signs are often late, not pathognomonic and represented by:

- a simple abdominal discomfort ;
- pelvic or abdominal pains;
- a progressive increase of abdominal volume due to a mass or ascites;
- bleeding and vaginal discharge;
- disorders of intestinal transit and symptoms of urinary irritations;
- more rarely, the signs of venous or radicular compression in the form of oedema of one lower limb, phlebitis or sciatica;
- a dyspnoea which may be in relation to a pleural effusion;
- a thoracic pain;
- a deterioration in the general health status.

A complete clinical and particularly gynaecological digital pelvic examinations, abdomen and lymph node areas palpation will help to identify a non-specific ovarian or pelvic mass. In this context, MRI, better than supra or endo-vaginal ultrasound and abdomino-pelvic CT scan is recommended to characterise any pelvic-tumour or lombo-aortic lymphadenopathies.

The dosage of tumoral markers such as CA-125, β HCG and alpha-fetoprotein can direct the tumour diagnoses especially those of germinal forms. It can also enable the assessment of the treatment quality and served as reference during the post-therapeutic follow-up.

Diagnosis of confirmation

The diagnosis of confirmation is only possible with the pathological examination of a biopsy sample done if possible by coelioscopic surgery. Nevertheless, it is most often obtained in our practice after laparotomy, followed by an analysis of the total tumour mass.

However, a guided needle aspiration echography can enable a cytology examination which, unfortunately, is only helpful with a relative assurance when positive.

Histological types

The various histologic types are represented:

- In more than 90% of the cases by epithelial cancers whose main sub-types are made up of serous, mucinous, endometrioïd forms, of clear, transitional, mixed, and undifferentiated cells.
- The mesenchymal forms with Leydig, Sertoli and lymphomatous cells are met in less than 10% of the cases.

III. Extension assessment of the tumour and the patient

- ***Extension assessment of the tumour***

Locally, it is to specify through a digital pelvic gynaecological examination, followed by an abdomino-pelvic echography or CT scan, the seat and volume of the primary tumour.

At the regional level, the stage of invasion of regional organs and pelvic lymph nodes will be assessed using echography, CT scan, and even better, the MRI.

At distance, the search for visceral metastases will be done mainly by imaging methods (standard radiography, echography, CT scan, MRI, PET/SCAN image fusion) directed if possible by symptomatology.

In case of pleural effusion or abdominal ascites, a puncture, with cytology of the liquid, can be used for the confirmation of a peritoneal carcinomatosis.

- ***Assessment of the patient***

By the clinical, imaging and biology examination, the general health status of the patient will be assessed by searching for particular cardiovascular, renal, metabolic and immunosuppression defects.

IV. Classification and prognostic factors

This classification is based according to the International Federation for Gynaecologists and Obstetricians (FIGO) on anatomo-clinical data.

Stages	Descriptions
Stage I	Tumour confined to the ovary
Stage IA	One affected ovary, intact capsule
Stage IB	Two affected ovaries, intact capsule
Stage IC	Ruptured capsule, neoplasic cells in the ascetic fluid or peritoneal washing
Stage II	Pelvic extension
Stage IIA	Extension to the uterus or fallopian tube
Stage II B	Extension to other pelvic organs
Stage II C	Visceral pelvic extension and neoplasic cells in the ascitic fluid or peritoneal washing
Stage III	Peritoneal extension out of the pelvis or lymph nodes metastases
Stage IIIA	Microscopic peritoneal localisations
Stage IIIB	Macroscopic peritoneal localisations < 2 cm
Stage IIIC	Peritoneal extension > 2 cm or lymph nodes localisations.
Stage IV	Distant visceral metastases excluding peritoneal localisations

V. Therapeutic means and methods

- ***The surgery***

It is about a loco regional method of a radical treatment whose technique comprises a total hysterectomy, a bilateral annexectomy, a complete omentectomy, an optional appendectomy for mucinous forms and finally a pelvic and lombo-aortic lymph node dissection passing through a broad supra, para and sub-umbilical laparotomy.

The surgical report must have information related to:

- The assessment of observed lesions, whose seat, size, morphological aspects will be specified.
- The description of the surgical acts carried out as well as the seat and dimensions of the tumoral after-effects that will be clipped.
- The sample for a cytological study of the ascitic fluid or peritoneal cleaning to the physiological solution.

- ***The chemotherapy***

It is about a loco regional and general method of treatment. The standard protocol is a poly-chemotherapy which generally associates carboplatin and paclitaxel.

A total of 6 cycles is parentally administered at the rate of a cycle every 21 days. The peritoneal route can be used in a particular case of peritoneal carcinomatosis.

- ***The radiotherapy***

It is also about a loco regional method of treatment, through ionising radiations, whose carrying out passes through a rigorous determination of irradiation parameters:

- Position of the patient during the treatment: the supine position is very often adopted for the reasons already above-mentioned;
- The target volume comprises the abdominal and pelvic cavity entirely;
- Total dose : it should not exceed for digestive tolerance reasons, the limit of 20-30 Gy provided according to the fractionation and traditional staggering of 5X2 Gy/ week thanks to the gamma radiation of 1,25 Mev, Cobalt 60 or rather X photons of 15-25 Mev of the Linear Accelerator;
- The projected computer-assisted dosimetry enables to improve the centring parameters and to optimise the distribution of the dose in the target volume.

VI. Indications and therapeutic protocols

Indications	Therapeutic protocols
Stage I and II - Epithelial or mesenchymal cancer - Good health in general	- First radical surgery - Radiotherapy (more or less)
Stage III and IV - Epithelial or mesenchymal cancer - Good health in general	- First chemotherapy - Surgery (in a second stage) - Radiotherapy in a third stage if tumoral after-effects < 2 cm
Stage I, II III IV - Lymphoma cancer	- First chemotherapy - Assessment in the second stage - Adapted surgery in the third stage - Radiotherapy in the fourth and last stage

VII. Results, Means and Methods of Follow-up

- ***Current results***

The prognosis of epithelial tumours is generally bad because of the importance of advanced forms.

The survival rate in 5 years without progressive disease is:

- 70 to 80% for well-differentiated stages I
- 15% for little differentiated stages III or II.

The prognosis is better for germinal tumours because of their high curability, chemo and radio sensitivity.

The cure of stages I with the fertility preservation of contro-lateral ovary is almost 100%.

For advanced stages, II III IV, the cure rate remains high around 70 to 80%.

For the supervision and post-therapeutic follow-up in short, medium and long term, appointments for consultation will be planned at least every 4 months for 2 years, and every 6 months for 3 years, then annually.

VIII. Prospects

Technical and budgetary measures will be taken to refine the diagnosis of ovarian cancers, through a systematic research for BRCA1 and BRCA2 antigenic markers; even if it is done despite all the difficulties, by means of an international collaboration through the sending of biopsy punch in the laboratories of the Northern countries.

Vulva cancers

I. Epidemiological specificities

Vulva cancer accounts for approximately 5% of genital cancers of the woman.

This cancer, very often affects the old woman with an average age of 67. However, it can be observed in developing countries like Cameroon from the age of 40.

Vulva cancer in 30% of cases at least, is multifocal of vulvar, vaginal and cervical seats at the same time.

The main pre-cancerous lesions of the vulva are represented by dystrophies, cancers in situ (Bowen's disease, Bowen's papulosis of the young woman) and giant condyloma acuminata. These lesions are sometimes diffuse, but remain superficial.

II. Diagnostic procedure

Inaugural symptomatology is poor, or unremarkable and consequently, very neglected. The functional signs are mainly: vulvar itch, noted in 30% of the patients; tumour, main sign in 50% of the patients; the bleeding and pain in 10%; urinary disorders in 5% and adenopathies in 2%.

The clinical examination and in particular the gynaecological one must be careful and supplemented if possible with a colposcopy enabling to carry out biopsies and histological examinations.

It is about:

- Squamous cell carcinoma in 90% of the cases.
- Basal cell carcinoma, melanoma and sarcoma being rare forms.

III. Extension assessment of the tumour and patient

- ***Extension assessment of the tumour***

The loco-regional extension assessment must take into account that, vulvar lymphatic routes are crossed and that: previous injuries, particularly clitoral ones have direct and pelvic draining paths.

Bilateral and iliac inguinal problems must systematically be searched for, by means of clinical examinations, ultrasound scan, tomodensitometry and especially MRI. In obese patients, the scan-directed cytoponction of inguinal adenopathies may sometimes be necessary to assert the diagnosis.

- ***Assessment of the patient***

The pre-therapeutic assessment in particular, the pre-surgical one must be exhaustive in order to search for, associated defects: diabetes, HTA, obesity, cardiac/renal insufficiency, trophic disorders and viral infections (HIV, Viral hepatitis A, B, C).

IV. Classification

TNM and FIGO classifications represented in the table below are the most used.

Stage TNM	Stage FIGO
T_1 <2 cm	I
T_2 >2 cm	II
T_3 Lower portion urethra/vagina/perineum/anus	III
T_4 Upper portion urethra/bladder/rectum/pelvis	IV
N_1 Unilateral/mobile lymph nodes	N1
N_2 Bilateral/mobile lymph nodes	N2
N_3Fixed lymph nodes	N3

V. Means and methods of treatment

- ***The surgery***

With a curative aim, it enables controlling the disease in its loco-regional development stage. The radical method necessary comprises a total vulvectomy associated with a bilateral inguinal cleaning out.

- ***The Radiotherapy***

It is about a loco-regional method of treatment with a curative aim, whose implementation passes through the rigorous determination of the main parameters of irradiation such as:

- The position of the patient during the treatment: The supine position ;
- The target volume very often comprises the vulva, inguinal nodal stations and pelvic ganglia;

- The total dose: it ranges from 65-70 Gy and is provided with a curative aim, according to the fractionation and traditional staggering of 5 times 2 Gy a week, thanks to the gamma radiation of an average energy of 1.25 MeV of cobalt 60 or X photons of 15 -25 MeV of the Linear Accelerator of Particles.

- ***The chemotherapy:***

It is about a loco-regional and general means of treatment, whose main protocol very often used in our environments, inter alia, for economic reasons is a chemotherapy policy comprising the 5-fluorouracil and Cisplatin.

VI. Indications and Therapeutic Protocols

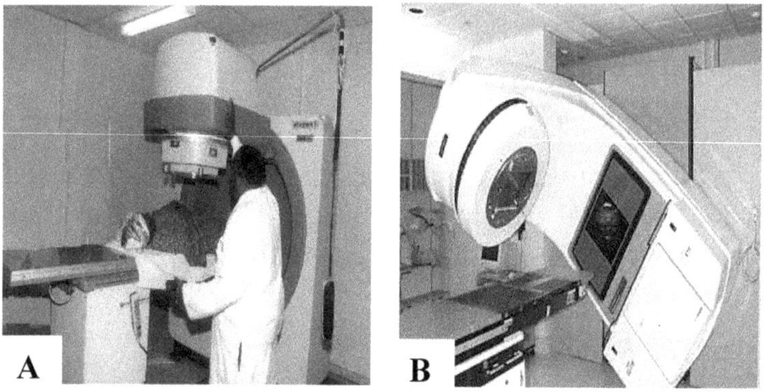

External Radiotherapy Machines
A : Cobalt 60 Machine (2D Radiotherapy at Yaounde General Hospital)
B : Linear Accelerator Machine (3D conformal Radiotherapy)

Indications	**Therapeutic protocols**
Stage T1 T2 : - Multifocal tumour - Good medical field	Radical surgery : Total vulvectomy plus Inguinal cleaning out D+G
Stage T1 T2 : - Old patients/ patients with a defect - Bad general state of health	Simple total vulvectomy, If palpable lymph nodes : biopsy + radiotherapy
T_3 T_4 - Good general state of health	First chemotherapy, Surgery in a second stage And radiotherapy in the third and last stage.
T_3 T_4 - Good general state of health - Advanced age	Exclusive radiotherapy

VII. Current results, means and methods of Follow-up

- ***Current results***

The best results in 5 years are obtained through the surgery

SR : 55 –75 % : in case of ideal surgery

SR : 30 –40 % : in case of unsatisfactory surgery

SR : 30 –60 % : Radio-surgical associations

SR: 20 –30% to 70 %(average 42%): Exclusive radiotherapy

The lymph node involvement is a major prognostic factor.

- ***Means and methods of follow-up:***

Consultations of supervision will be planned in short, medium and long term, with an aim at assessing therapeutic results, searching for recurrences and treating them. Clinical, gynaecological examinations and Pap smear on one hand; then, both imaging (CT and MRI) will be an essential contribution.

Indeed, complications are frequent. In immediate post-surgical can occur a division of the surgical wound, a lymphorragy and flap necrosis.

Oedema of lower limbs, curable hernias, an incontinence and a urinary prolapse will represent the main late complications.

VIII. Preventive measures and prospects

- The primary and secondary prevention in particular for young people will mainly be based on the dietary education, the research and treatment of pre-cancerous lesions.
- The improvement of the current results in particular for the advanced stages III and IV that are the most frequent in our hospital environments is possible through the contribution and access of all the patients to chemotherapy with more effective molecules.
- At the surgical level, human, technological and organisational measures should be taken for the development of the reconstructive surgery.

PART TWO

UROLOGICAL CANCERS

Prostate cancers

I. Epidemiological specificities

In the West as in Africa, the frequency of prostate cancer is growing gradually. The average age of occurrence is around 65 in the Northern countries. It is even lower in Cameroon and ranges from 40 to 50, where its prognosis is poorer in 90% of the patients at the late stages.

The etiological factors are mainly genetic (the black race is more affected), hormonal and infectious (chronic prostatitis).

II. Diagnostic procedure

In anamnestic terms, the more or less early symptoms are urinary in the form of frequent micturition (especially at night-time), reduction in the stream of urine, feeling of incomplete emptying of the urine bladder, total and brutal impossibility to urinate (acute urine retention) and a mass at the lower abdomen (vesical globe).

The late symptoms rather rectal in the form of constipation by rectal and bone tumoral compression with lombo-pelvic pains and paralysis of the limbs following the pathological fractures and medullary compression.

The biological approach of the diagnosis of prostate cancer is particularly based on the PSA test, whose any increase in the rate is strongly predictive of a tumoral problem likely to be malignant or benign.

In this context, the digital rectal exam (DRE), especially when it is echo- guided, remains through its very great sensitivity, the best clinical means unanimously recognised to search for the signs of an intra-prostatic tumoral presence that may result in an increase in the prostate volume, the existence of one or several nodules in a lobe, the filling of the median fissure or an irregularity with unclear limit of prostatic contour.

The ultrasound imaging, in particular the transrectal one, is particularly recommended and sufficient to confirm the signs obtained with the DRE.

The diagnosis of certainty is exclusively histologic and is obtained after echo-guided biopsy or tumour trans-urethral resection and anatomopathological study of the part obtained.

Adenocarcinoma is the most frequent histologic type of which the degrees of differentiation expressed in Gleason score: GI, GII, GIII are correlated with the prognosis, in particular, metastatic: good, intermediate and bad in this order.

III. Extension assessment of the tumour and the patient

- ***Extension assessment of the tumour***

The aim of the assessment of local extension is to specify the seat of the primary tumour and its size or volume using the RDE and endo-rectal ultrasound scan, both, by clinical and para clinical means very accessible and sensitive, which will give the precise details on the seat as well as the number and volume of the nodules and prostate, information on the importance of the micturition residue.

The assessment of the level of regional extension of the primary tumour will be done through the research of the close organs invasion and especially for pelvic nodal stations.

To be done, the means of imaging usually used nowadays, in our hospitals environments like ultrasound scan and tomodensitometry, are unfortunately not very sensitive and less effective in particular for the research of the ganglia, for economic reasons.

The high cost and limited access of the MRI as well as a total absence of the techniques of image fusion: Scan/Tep with 18FDG, more recommended, sensitive and efficient significantly contribute to limiting the relevance of the extension assessments and by extension, the quality of therapeutic results in low-income countries.

Coelio-surgery is an optional method of regional extension assessment. It still remains very little practised in our hospitals for budgetary shortfall reasons. However, it is a little invasive and very contributory surgical technique in terms of surgical histologic study of ganglia, assessment of ganglionic extension itself and the treatment through ilio-obturator lymphadenectomy.

The distant assessment of tumoral extension will be done through the search for visceral and mainly bone metastases. In addition to the usual clinical means, we will use the imaging, which will be as far as possible directed by symptomatology for economic reasons and effectiveness. According to the cases and technical facilities, a chest X-ray will be prescribed, an abdomino-pelvic ultrasound scan, a scan or abdomino-pelvic or brain MRI entirely and if possible a bone scintigraphy.

- ***Pre-therapeutic assessment of the patient***

The aim of the pre-therapeutic assessment is to assess using specific clinical, radiological and biological examinations and if possible a bone scan, the general state of health of the patient and to search for defects such as: cardiac, renal, pulmonary and immunological problems.

IV. Classification and prognostic factors

- ***Prognostic factors and degrees of severity***

Prognostic factors	**Good prognoses**	**Intermediate prognoses**	**Bad prognoses**
TNM	T0, T1, small T2, N0, M0	Big T2, N0, M0	T3, T4, N2, N3, N+, M+
Gleason score	GI	GII	GIII
PSA level	< 10 ng/ml (1/3 extracapsular cancers)	Level between 10 and 20 ng/ml (a capsular overrun or a probable ganglion invasion)	> 30 ng/ml, presence of bone metastasis in 85% of the cases with pathological bone scan or spread ganglionic waiting if negative metastatic assessment
Analysis of the surgical part	• Healthy resection margins • Absence of capsular overrun • Histologically healthy seminal vesicle • Histologically healthy ganglia (N-)		• Focally invasive resection margins • Existence of capsular overrun • Histologically affected seminal vesicle • Histologically affected ganglia (N+)
General state of the patient	Good general state (absence of defects)		General bad state (presence of defects)

- ***TNM Classification***

It is based on anatomo-clinical and histo-pathological data.

TNM	Description	Code US
T1	Chance discovery on adenomectomy part	**A**
T1a	< 3 seats	**A1**
T1b	> 3 seats	**A2**
T2	Palpable clinical tumour, limited to the gland	**B**
T2a	<1,5 cm	**B1**
T2b	>1,5 cm	**B2**
T3	Invasion of prostatic apex, capsular crossing, extension at the vesical neck or seminal vesicle, but without fixation	**C, C1, C2**
T4	Attached tumour or invasing the close structures	**C2**
N1	Unique adenopathy < 2 cm	**D1**
N2	Unique adenopathy >2 cm but < 5 cm, or many < 5 cm	**D1**
N3	Adenopathy > 5cm	**D1**
M1	Visceral metastases	**D2**

V. Methods and techniques of treatment

- ***External radiotherapy***

It is defined as a loco-regional method of treatment with a curative aim limited to the primary tumour and its pelvic lymph nodes extensions.

With a palliative aim, it will enable to relieve and to improve the comfort of the patient through an action on remote metastases.

- **Practical details and main techniques of external radiotherapy at Yaounde General Hospital (1987-2012)**

Radiotherapy machines	**Availability**	**Fx energy**	**Beam nature**	**Conformation**	**Total dose**	**IMRT**	**Tolerance**	**Results**
Co60	YES	1.25 MeV	Gamma-ray	2D	65-70 Gy	Non possible	medium	medium
Linear Accelerator	NO	25 MeV	X photons Electron	3D	Higher 70-80 Gy	possible	better	Better

- ***The Interstitial brachytherapy***

It is an optional technique recommended for curative treatment of tumours whose extension is strictly limited to the prostate, without any invasion of the lymph nodes and no metastases. Early stages: T1; T2; N0; M0.

The target volume is consequently very reduced; therefore, an excellent tolerance of irradiation and better therapeutic results.

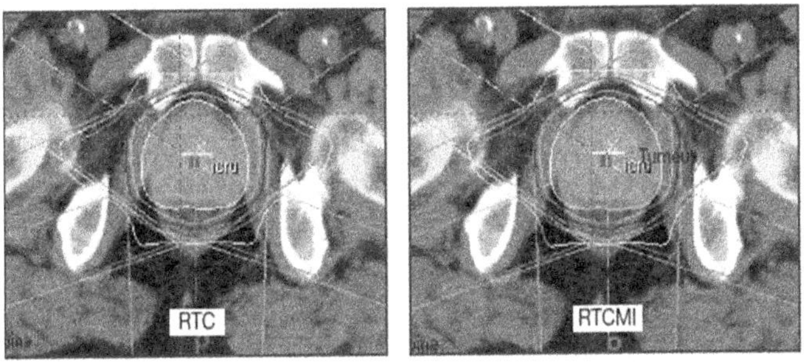

3D Dosimetry
RTC : Conformational Radiotherapy
RTCMI: Intensity Modulation Conformational Radiotherapy

- ***The surgery***

It is about a radical loco-regional method of treatment whose technique comprises a first ilio-obturating lymphadenectomy, followed by a radical prostatectomy through a supra pubic route if the lymph nodes are histologically healthy.

- ***The hormone therapy***

This method will act on the local, regional and general level at the same time.

Its aim is to obtain an androgenic suppression, therefore to limit tumoral growth.

The protocol of first line includes: a pulpectomy, a chemical castration by the LH-RH agonists and a complete androgenic blocking: Anti-Androgen+Castration

- ***The chemotherapy***

Like hormone therapy, chemotherapy is also a loco-regional and general method of treatment of cancers even of prostatic origin.

However, it is unfortunately, little active, badly adapted in the field. There is not any protocol of reference, and is only recommended in case of hormone-resistance in the young person.

VI. Indications and treatment protocols

STAGES	THERAPEUTIC STRATEGIES	NUMBER OF TREATED PATIENTS (HGY experience) 2012
T_{1a} (Gleason bas; advanced age)	Therapeutic abstention and strict follow up	No patient (0 %)
T_{1b}-T_{1c}-T_2	- Two options of equal value - Radical surgery - Exlusive radiotherapy	1/85(2%)
T_{1b}-T_{1c}-T_2 R+ Seminal vesicle seminal +N-/+ Normal PSA	Surgery + radiotherapy	No patient (0 %)
T_3 N-M-	Exclusive radiotherapy	2/85 (3 %)
T_3 N+M+	Hormone therapy	30/85(36%)
T_4M+	Palliative (antalgic and decompression)	52/85 (62 %)

- ***Current results***

SR without recurrence	**5 years**		**10 years**	
Stages	Literature	Our series	Literature	Our series
T1	85%	0%	75%	0%
T2	65%	0%	50%	0%
T3	50%	0%	30%	0%

VII. Means and methods of follow-up

Consultations will be planned and organised in short, medium and long terms to assess therapeutic results thanks to suitable clinical, biological and radiological examinations, and to search for loco-regional and general recurrences as well as complications or iatrogenic after-effects, whose care is necessary for the family and socio-professional reintegration.

VIII. Simple methods of early diagnosis and prospects.

The significant improvement of the current results in Cameroon will be effective only through an organisation of awareness and early screening campaigns by the proportion of PSA test and early diagnosis by the TR of the target populations in particular from 45.

At the therapeutic level, it will be necessary to make the most effective drugs available in the resistant forms to the hormone therapy and to develop better imaging techniques of extension assessment and treatment through conformational radiotherapy, irradiation in intensity modulation and dosimetry 3D.

Bladder cancers

I. Epidemiological specificities

Apart from certain countries of the Maghreb such as Egypt, in Africa in general and particularly in Cameroon, data on the frequency of bladder cancers are imprecise and far from being pathognomonic. However, its scarcity is much more admitted, except in areas of endemic of Schistosoma haematobium bilharzian diseases. The most incriminated etiological factors are: tobacco addiction, chronic bladder infections, and bladder lithiasis. But chemical components such as: pesticides, herbicides, aniline and other substances of the same nature, have been since known in the West and in Africa only during these last decades, to be bladder carcinogenic. The increasingly use of these chemicals, especially in the agricultural activities, would be the cause of a progressive increase in the frequency of this cancer over the recent years in the world.

The average age of occurrence of bladder cancers is about 65. It may be less than 40 in case of bilharzian etiology. The sex-ratio is 3 men for a woman.

The most frequent inaugural symptomatology is mainly intermittent macroscopic hematuria. Suprapubic bladder pains with dysuria are less frequent, but become more severe with loco-regional tumour evolution.

II. Diagnostic Procedure

The early diagnosis is based on an endoscopic exploration in case of microscopic or macroscopic hematuria:

- The cystoscopy will permit to specify the seat of the primary tumour at the mobile and fixed portion of the bladder in 60 % to 40 % of the cases respectively; the lateral faces being frequently the focal area of multi-site or diffuse disease of urothelium. The tumoral biopsy will be done during the cystoscopy for a histologic diagnosis:
  - Non infiltrating papillary tumour but nevertheless, with a strict local recurrence tendency in 50 to 60 % of the cases for 10 years. The evolution to an invasive cancer can be observed in 8 to 12 % of the cases. The survival rate in 10 years is 90 %.
  - Carcinoma in situ may become invasive cancer after 5 or 7 years in 50 to 70 % of the cases.
  - Invasive cancers are most often multifocal, invasive zones may surround in situ or dysphasic ones. But cases of isolated or uni focal tumour may exist.
- Urinary cytology is recommended for its specificity and sensitivity, especially in case of carcinoma *in situ.*

- The anatomopathological study of the surgical specimen will enable to evaluate the level of penetration in the bladder wall which progresses in stages: chorion-muscle-peri vesical fat and close organs. The lymphatic extension accelerates with the volume of the tumour and the degree of penetration in the bladder wall. External iliac, hypogastric, primary and lombo-aortic lymph nodes are gradually affected in this order.

Metastases are mainly bony, pulmonary or hepatic ones.

III. Extension assessment of the tumour and the patient

- ***Tumoral extension assessment***

The implementation of this assessment will be rigorous and exhaustive at the local level to determine the site and volume of the primary tumour to estimate the degree of invasion of close organs and pelvic lymph nodes at the regional level; and finally at a distance, the search for visceral metastases, very often in lungs, bones and liver. To reach this important objective, whose impact on the treatment is well established, it is recommended to use only very well proved sensitive and specific methods of examination, even though there are not available for obvious reasons in our hospital milieu.

a) Therefore, at the local level:

- The digital rectal examination associated to bimanual palpation will permit, with a bit application, to reach the set objectives and even to specify the degree of parietal penetration and the unique or multiple characters of the lesions.
- Intravenous urography may be normal even in the presence of obvious infiltrating cancer:
    - an unspecified bladder area can be the sign of a tumour;
    - uretero-pyelocalicial dilatation is often a sign of a muscle infiltration or a second tumour on the ureter or the renal pelvis;
- once more, cystoscopy will permit a significant contribution especially in case of doubt of a normal

urography with the presence of an obvious infiltrating cancer.

b) At the regional level:

- Echography, CT scan have limited values, particularly for the diagnosis of lymph nodes invasion with false-positive in 50 % of the cases.
- Coelio surgery, if applicable will enable to refine the diagnosis by correcting the false-positive of the scanner, but also to assess the tumour extension and to start the treatment with an external iliac lymphadenectomy.
- MRI, in spite of its limited accessibility, is the most recommended examination technique for its sensitivity and specificity.

c) At distance, the search for visceral metastases will be done according to the localisations and quality of the available technical facilities, by:

- Clinical and radiological means as chest or bone segment standard radiography, thoraco-abdomino-pelvic echography, cerebral CT scan and bone scintigraphy guided as far as possible by symptomatology in our hospital milieu, for economic and effictiveness reasons.

- ***Assessment of the patient***

Indeed, it is an operability assessment which aims is to evaluate the general status of the patient and to search for defects such as cardiovascular, hepatorenal, metabolic and immunological ones using suitable clinical, para-clinical and biological examinations.

IV. Classification and prognostic factors

- ***Histological prognostic factors:***

Histological prognostic factors	**Severity parameters**
Non infiltrating papillary tumours	High risk of local relapse if : -multiple site character -size>1cm -degree of differenciation WHO>2
Carcinoma *in situ*	Risk of evolution for a possible infiltration
Infiltrating Cancers	vital risk: if local and metastatic evolution particularly in case of sessile tumour or diameter >5 cm
Other factors of aggravation, and poor prognoses	Site on the fixed portion of the bladder, Multifocal character Degree of penetration into the wall. Important and massive lymph node involvement, Inoperability of a tumour and the absence of a response at the neoadjuvant radiotherapy

- ***TNM classification***

Tis	Carcinoma in situ
Ta	Non-invasive papillary carcinoma
T1	Sub-epithelial connective tissue tumour invasion
T2	Inner halth of superficial muscle tumour invasion
T3	Deep muscle (T3a) or peri-vesical fat (T3b) tumour invasion
T4	One or more surronding organs tumour invasion : prostate, uterus, vagina, abdominal or pelvic walls
N0	No metastatic regional adenopathy
N1	Unique adenopathy < 2cm
N2	Unique Metastasis >2 cm and >5 cm or multiple all < 5 cm
N3	Lymph node metastasis >5 cm

V. Therapeutic means and methods

- ***The surgery***

The surgery is the reference treatment for invasive bladder cancers. Three techniques are currently used depending on the case:

- Trans-urethral endoscopic resection (TUR). It is used both as therapeutic and diagnostic means with a histologic study of the specimen resection. It is known as a tumoral reduction surgery with a poor carcinological result but nevertheless, should be complete as far as possible.

- Partial cystectomy. The first step consists in verifying on frozen section biopsy, the absence of lymph node invasion. Then, the second step which leads to the total resection of the tumour including a safety margin.
- Total cystectomy. It is a very heavy operation which most often consist of a cysto-prostatectomy in men and an anterior pelvectomy, with hysterectomy in women pre-justified by an ilio-obturator lymphadenectomy, with non-invasive lymph node histology study. This surgical protocol requires the urine derivation according to several techniques :
  - trans-intestinal cutaneous derivation of Bricker's type more frequently used;
  - bilateral cutaneous ureterostomy often indicated for the most fragile patients;
- entero-cystoplasty recommended for men only when the external sphincter of the ureter has been preserved.

▪ ***The radiotherapy***

Two techniques are used:

- The external radiotherapy, defined as such because the radioactive source which produces the radiation is placed outside and at a certain distance from the patient. Its implementation requires the determination of all irradiation parameters of which the main ones are:
  - The position of the patient on the treatment machine: the supine position is very often adopted for its simplicity, the patient comfort and especially the reproducibility accuracy all over the treatment time.

- The target volume: it includes the entire pelvis with the bladder and all external and internal iliac lymph nodes.
- The total dose: it ranges from 45-65 Gy in case of indication of an adjuvant radiotherapy after incomplete surgery or exclusive radiotherapy.

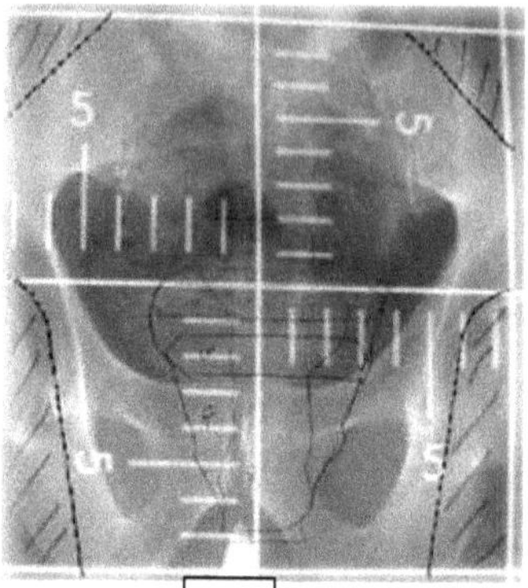

A

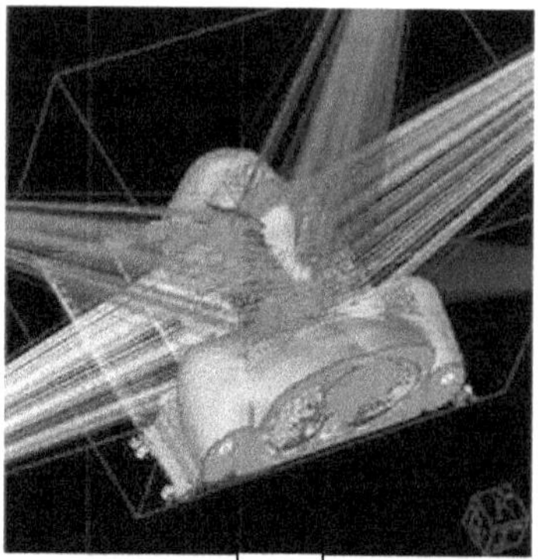

B

External Radiotherapy techniques

A : 2D DSA Simulation technique using two opposed fields (01 anterior/01 posterior)

B : 3D Multifields Conformational Simulation technique

- The interstitial brachytherapy or endo-brachytherapy: in this technique, the radioactive source is rather directly inserted within the tumour, the resection margins with a low-value carcinological surgery.

- ***The chemotherapy:***

The systematic method remains the most used after a gradual abandonment of intra-vesical administration of Doxorubicin, Mitomycin or BCG. The most effective protocols are MVAC and CMV, made up of: Methotrexate, Velbe, Adriblastine and Cyclophosphamide.

VI. Indications and therapeutic protocols

Indications	Therapeutic protocols
Ta	
Non infiltrating superficial papillary Cancers	Conservative treatment : iterative Trans Urethral Resection (TUR) or Electrocoagulation
If recurrence	Repeated endo- vesical instillations : Adriamycin+THIOTH EPA +MITOMYCIN C : once/week for 6 weeks or BCG
Tis	Total cystectomy at once
T1	
T1<4 cm : unique tumour mainly papillary no CIS nor associated dysplasia	TUR + follow-up + local instillation
If multiple recurrence	Total or partial cystectomy + Brachytherapy
T2	Conservative treatment close to T1 or radical attitude as in T3
T3	1st ERT surgery Adjuvant ERT
T3 3a 3b	1st concomitant radio-chemotherapy + radical surgery or exclusive radiotherapy. In case of surgical or general contraindication
T4	Palliative Radiotherapy : 20 Gy/5f/5Days
M+	Chemotherapy protocol : MVAC

VII. Current results

- Superficial Cancers: cure rate in 5 years: 90 %
- Invasive Cancers : 60-80 %
    - If exclusive RT: 20-30 %
    - If Metastasis: lower than 10 %

VIII. Preventive measures and prospects

- Primary preventive measures must be systematically taught at the individual level during the consultation of the patient, and at the level of the target population, during mass educational campaigns for a behaviour change in particular: tobacco, pesticides, infectious and parasitic risks.
- Secondary preventive measures will be focused on the screening and treatment of precancerous lesions during mass campaigns.
- A significant improvement of the current therapeutic results will be possible only by means of an innovation of early diagnosis, extension assessment and treatment. The implementation of more effective chemotherapy protocols is particularly recommended at first line for our patients, whose over 75% arrive at advanced stages.

Renal cancers

I. Epidemiological specificities

Renal cancer affects men twice more than women. The average age at the diagnosis ranges from 55 to 60.

In Cameroon, renal cancers represent 1 % of all cancers observed within the general population and ranked 16th in the list of all cancers.

The factors of renal carcinogenesis are poorly known, except tobacco addiction, chronic renal lithiasis and the dialysis treatment for over three years.

II. Diagnostic Procedure

The most relatively early signs and symptoms observed are represented by a unilateral or bilateral lumbar mass, hematuria, lumbago and an unknown origin fever. Other late, varied and less specific signs and symptoms may appear under the form of a simple discomfort or abdominal pains, or a progressive abdominal increase in the volume, due to a mass or rarely ascites, mictional disorder with dysuria, pollakiuria and urinary urgency, an abdominal syndrome compression with transit disorder, sub-occlusion and false needs. More rarely, a venous or radicular syndrome compression with oedema of a lower limb, phlebitis or sciatalgia. Finally, a chest pain, a dyspnoea, or a deterioration of the general status may be related to a metastatic development, particularly of pleuropulmonary type.

However, it is relevant to note that renal cancer may be observed in the absence of any sign and symptom, during a systematic examination with abdominal echography or CT scan, without any specific aims.

Unfortunately, most often, for economic reasons, this cancer is fortuitously discovered in very late stages with abdominal metastases and neoplastic poly adenopathies in our hospital environments. The clinical examination enables to palpate in 20 % of the cases, a lumbar or abdominal mass, which is easily confirmed by abdominal echography or CT scan.

The final step of diagnosis confirmation is by histology after the anatomopathological examination of the biopsy specimen or as often in disadvantaged environments, the total tumour sample after radical surgery for both diagnostic and therapeutic aims.

In developed countries, 90 % of adult renal cancers are clear cells carcinomas or chromophobe also called renal cell carcinoma or Grawitz's tumour.

In developing countries, in children, nephroblastoma is observed in 75 %, carcinomas in 20 % and Burkitt's lymphoma in 5 % of the cases respectively.

Nephoblastoma or Wilms' tumour, the child's tumour, as well as 2 to 3 % of renal cancers of genetic origin will be developed in a specific book.

III. Extension assessment of the tumour and the patient

- ***Extension assessment of the tumour:***

Before any treatment, in particular, surgical one, it is relevant to study:

- The local extension of the primary, unique or multiple tumour, located in a pole, perhaps still limited by the capsule or renal fossa invasion of contralateral kidney.
- The regional extension of the primary tumour within surronding organs, starting from the renal fossa, the psoas muscles and adrenal gland; then in abdomino-pelvic lymph nodes, the homolateral renal vein and the inferior vena cava.
- The distance metastatic extension of the primary tumour must be systematically searched at the level of adrenal gland, contralateral kidney, lungs, bones, liver and the brain.

The suitable means of the tumour extension assessment in all progressive steps are on the base of the performance of technical diagnostic means constituted besides clinical examinations, by CT scan and MRI which are nknown much more effective and sensitive than echography, which is unfortunately very often used in our hospital environments for economic reasons.

For the same economic reasons, the echo-doppler and MRI are very rarely prescribed and implemented in our milieu with the indication to estimate the level of extension of the tumour in the inferior vena cava and even until the right cardiac atrium even if the theurapetic interests of this assessment is well known.

- ***Assessment of the patient***

The objective of this assessment is to evaluate using clinical, biological and radiological methods, the general status of the patient, then, search for defects which may be cardiovascular, renal, metabolic, hypertensive or immunodepressive.

IV. Classification and prognostic factors

- ***Prognostic factors***

Considering the major role of surgery in the therapeutic care, the distinction of operable forms of good prognosis from inoperable ones of poor prognosis is possible and useful on the base of the anatomo-clinical extension assessment data of the tumour and the patient.

- ***TNM and Robson classification***

It is based on clinical and radiological initial data; then, on post-surgical findings and the result of the anatomopathological examination of the surgical specimen.

TNM classification		**ROBSON classification**	
Indications	**Description**	**Indications**	**Description**
T0	Absence of tumour		
T1	Tumour < to 2,5 cm	TI	Tumour confined in parenchyma ; capsule intact
T2	Tumour > to 2,5 cm, confined in the kidney	TII	Extension to the peri-renale fat or to the excretory tract
T3a	Invasion of adrenal gland or peri-renal fat	TIIIA	Involvement of the renal vein and inferior vena cava
T3b	Invasion of main renal vein or	TIIIB	Lymph node involvement

	subdiaphragmatic inferior vena cava		
T3c	Susdiaphragmatic inferior vena cava	TIIIC	veinous and lymph node involvement
T4	Above renale fossa	TIVA	Extension to surrounding organs
		TIVB	Metastases
NX	Unspecified		
N0	No lymph node involvement		
N1	A regional lymph node < to 2 cm		
N2	A regional lymph node > 2 cm and < 5 cm or several lymph nodes < to 5 cm		
N3	A regional lymph node superior to 5 cm		
MX	Unspecified		
M0	Absent		
M1	Positive		

V. Means and methods of treatment

- ***The surgery***

The surgery is the main curative treatment whose technique includes a broad total nephrectomy removing the kidney, the renal fossa, adrenal gland and regional juxta-hilary and latero-aortic lymph nodes.

The thrombectomy of a thrombus located within the renal vein or inferior vena cava is sometimes necessary and does not make the prognosis worse.

- ***Arterial embolisation***

Arterial embolisation is sometimes indicated and useful in pre-surgical protocol to limit bleeding in case of very vascularised primary tumour and metastases. It also has an antalgic interest in case of surgical contraindications.

- ***Ablation by radio frequency and heat or cryoablation***

None of these techniques is yet available in our hospital environments, even if their interest is demonstrated in case of partial surgery with the preservation of the function of the kidney after tumour ablation.

- ***The Radiotherapy***

It is mainly a tele-radiotherapy that may be curative or palliative, whose implementation needs the determination of the main irradiation parameters which are:

- The position of the patient on the treatment machine: the supine position is very often adopted for its simplicity, the patient comfort and especially the reproducibility accuracy all over the treatment time.
- The target volume to be irradiated, generally the renal fossa and lymph node areas.
- The total dose: it ranges from 45-50 Gy and provided by ɣ -radiation of an average energy of 1.25 MeV of cobalt 60 or X- radiation of an average energy of 15-25 MeV of the linear accelerator of particles.

- The computer-assisted pre-treatment dosimetry, whose role in the improvement of the quality and tolerance of the irradiation is not to be demonstrated any more.

- ***The chemotherapy***

Because of its low effectiveness, chemotherapy is only indicated for research prospective protocol and evaluation.

VI. Indications and therapeutic protocols

Indications	**Therapeutic protocol**
Stage T_1 $T_2T_3T_4$ $N_0N_1N_2N_3M_0$ Operable patient	Radical surgery: large total nephrectomy removing the kidney, renal fossa, adrenal gland and regional juxta-hilary and latero-aortic lymph nodes
Stage T_1 $T_2T_3T_4$ $N_0N_1N_2N_3M_0$ Incomplete surgery	Eternal radiotherapy : 45-50 Gy : 5x2Gy/week
Stage T_1 $T_2T_3T_4$ $N_0N_1N_2N_3M_0$ Inoperable patient	Treatment with a palliative aim: Radiotherapy 30 Gy / 10f / 12 days Chemotherapy Immunotherapy
M+	Treatment with a palliative aim: Radiotherapy 30 Gy / 10f/ 12 days Chemotherapy Immunotherapy

VII. Current results and follow-up

- ***Follow-up***

Follow-up consultations will be scheduled and organised in short, medium and long terms, every 4 months for 2 years, then, once yearly for 5 years at least. The aim is to confirm the positive results at the end of the treatment and to search for remote, local and regional recurrence without forgetting the complications or iatrogenic sequelae.

For that aim, clinical, radiological and biological methods of examinations will be used according to the case and guided as far as possible by symptomatology.

- ***Current results***

In general, adult renal cancers have a very good prognosis when the diagnosis is early and the proper treatment immediately applied. Unfortunately, it is not always the case in developing countries like Cameroon, where almost 80 % of patients arrive at late stages when only a palliative treatment remains possible.

Indeed, curative treatments are characterised by the following results:

5 years survival rate for 5 years :

- localised renal forms of N- : > 90 %
- Peri-renal fat extension forms:70 %
- N + form : 40 %
- Metastatic Forms: <10%

Prospects

- Develop at least one specialised screening centre of the populations at risk particularly those with family members concerned by a hereditary renal cancer
- Improve the quality of conservative treatments, with the introduction of radio frequency or cryoablation techniques.
- Moreover, the conception of a more effective chemotherapy and immunotherapy protocol would enable better care of operable and metastatic forms.

Testicular cancers

I. Epidemiological specificities

Testicular tumours are rare. They are rarer in black than white people with an annual incidence estimated at 2 or 3 for 100, 000 men and rank, first of all, cancers for the age groups between 21 and 35. They represent less than 1 % of male cancers in Cameroon.

Testicular atrophy following cryptorchidy remains the main known etiological factor. However, trauma and especially chronic testicular infections, seem to have a significant role in the origin of this cancer in our environments.

II. Diagnostic procedure

Swelling or testicular mass, often painless, is the revealing symptom or sign in more than 60 % of the cases. Therefore, it is the cause of late diagnosis in many cases, where metastatic extension is in the form of a painful abdominal tumour, sub-clavicular adenopathy or general asthenia syndrome. A gynaecomastia may be inaugural as sign of endocrine syndrome, with a gonadotrophin secretion.

On the clinical examination, the palpation of any testicular nodule must be considered as a cancer sign until histologically proven. Indeed, they do exist a certain number of differential diagnoses which are to be eliminated, most often after a comparative echography of both testicles: prolapsed hernia hydrocele, varicocele, orchitis and epididymis cyst.

The dosage in the blood of the general circulation and the spermatic vein of the main tumoral markers as alpha-foetoproteine, ß HCG and LDH, must be done before any surgical intervention with a guided and confirmed diagnostic aim. Moreover, these markers dosage will permit the evaluation of the therapeutic results.

Indeed, after orchidectomy, the fall of the rate of markers is often dramatic and fast, the biological half-life of Alfa-foetoproteine being five days and that of Beta HCG from 18 to 24 hours. Only the existence of a tumoral residue outside the removed testicle can explain a slower decrease of these markers. However, 10 % of pure seminoma presents a moderately high rate of BetaH CG but never Alfa-foetoproteine. Lastly, LDH is a non-specific marker of germinal tumours.

The diagnosis of testicular cancer can be confirmed only after histologic examination of the whole orchidectomy specimen after surgery carried out by high or inguinal route.

- ***Histological Classification of testicular tumours***

1- Germinal Tumours (GT): 95% of testicular tumours

1.1- Pure seminoma tumours (ST) : 35% of GT that are observed in men of 30 to 40 years old

1.2- Non seminoma tumours (NST) : 65 % of GT observed in men of 20 to 25 years old

Increase of ß HCG in 40 to 60% of the cases and alpha- fetoprotein in 70 % of the cases, if any existence of an embryonic carcinoma component.

2- Non Germinal Tumours (NGT) : 5% of testicular tumours

III. Assessment of tumoral extension

This assessment must be rigorous because of its prognostic and therapeutic impact:

- Locally: the site and volume of the primary tumour will be specified by the clinical examination and testicular echography;
- Regionally and at distance: the search for lymph nodes and visceral metastases mainly under the diaphragm (lombo-aortic) or upper the diaphragme (mediastinal and left sub-clavicular) is based on abdomino-pelvic and chest CT scan, then, the dosage of tumoral markers which has a diagnostic, therapeutic and follow-up importance.

IV. Assessment of the patient

It consists in:

- estimating the general status of the patient, the search for defects especially anatomo-clinical, biological and metabolic ones.
- collecting before any therapeutic act, the sperm for cryo-preservation in bank if its quality is confirmed. This technique of preservation of the possibilities of post-therapeutic reproduction, unfortunately, still remains unavailable in our hospital environments.

- ***Classification by anatomo-clinical stages***

It is better adapted than the TNM classification to the prognosis assessment and therapeutic orientation

- Stage I : tumour confined in the testicle
- Stage II : lombo-aortic lymph nodes metastases

  A : ≤ 2 cm in diameter

B : 2 to 5 cm in diameter

C : > 5 cm in diameter

- Stage III : Sus-diaphragmatic lymph nodes metastases
- Stage IV : visceral metastases

- ***Prognostic factors***

Factors of poor prognosis:
- More than 10 metastases per lung
- Presence of hepatic and cerebral metastases
- Palpable abdominal mass
- Important increase in tumoral markers

V. Therapeutic methods and techniques

- ***The surgery***

A testicular biopsy or even a minimal orchidectomy by a scrotal route is to be banned, for, it is carcinologically invalid and dangerous as the main origin of rapid loco-regional dissemination.

The large orchidectomy by a high, inguinal route remains the best surgical technique able to ensure the control, the tying and complete resection of the tumour and spermatic cord in one surgical operation.

The retro-peritoneal lymphadenectomy is no more systematically done as the first option in case of macroscopic lymph nodes invasion, because of the effectiveness of chemotherapy.

The exeresis of retro-peritoneal or pulmonary residual masses after chemotherapy may be recommended in case of partial response and if the tumoral markers are normal.

- ***The radiotherapy***

The parameters of irradiation must be determined with exactitude on the base of anatomo-clinical and extension assessment data:

➢ *The target volume (TV)*

- The sub-diaphragmatic TV includes: the lombo-aortic, homolateral, primitive iliac and external iliac lymph nodes.
- The sus-diaphragmatic target volume includes: the sub-clavicular and mediastinal lymph nodes effectively affected.

The inguino-scrotal target volume is no longer systematically treated, except in case of the anterior surgical treatment of inguino-scrotal hernia, hydrocele, trans-scrotal biopsy or orchidopexy.

➢ *The total dose*

It ranges according to the stage:

- Stage I : 20 to 25 Gray
- Stage IIa and IIb: 30 to 35 Gray more or less 5 to 10 Gray boost in the involved lymph nodes.

- ***The chemotherapy***

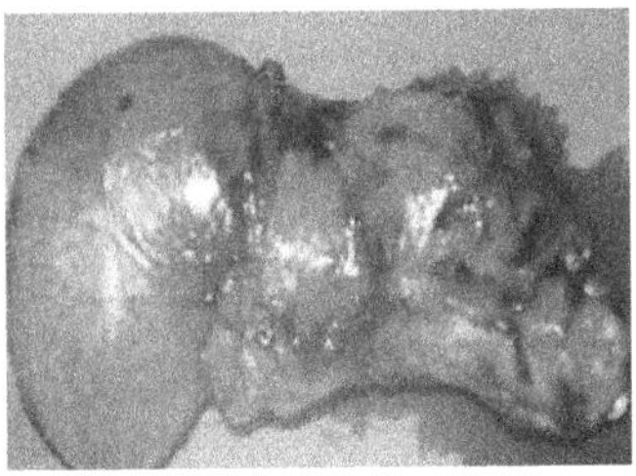

A

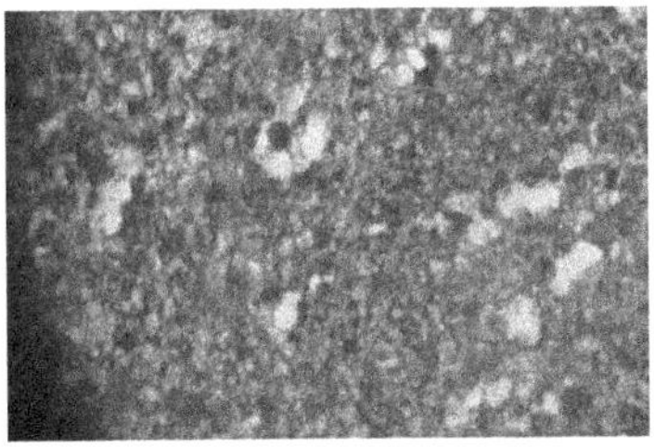

B

Burkitt Testicular Lymphoma

A : macroscopic specimen after an upper inguinal orchidectomy

B : specific histologic aspect with Giemsa technique

The main protocols recommended include: Cis-platin, Bleomycin, Vinblastine or Vepeside. Two are usually used:

- BEP (Bleomycin-Vepeside-Cisplatin) for good prognosis forms.
- PVeVB (4 drugs associated) for poor prognosis forms.

VI. Therapeutic Indications

They depend on the histologic type and the stage

<table>
<tr><th>Stages / Histology</th><th>I</th><th>IIA & IIB</th><th>IIC - IV</th></tr>
<tr><td>Seminoma</td><td>Prophylactic Radiotherapy</td><td>Curative radiotherapy</td><td>Chemotherapy
↓
partial or complete response
1 : simple follow-up
2 : radiotherapy
3 : exeresis of residual masses</td></tr>
<tr><td>non seminoma tumours</td><td>1 : Strict follow-up and chemotherapy in relapse cases
2: prophylactic retro-peritoneal lymphadenectomy and follow-up if healthy lymph nodes (N-)
3 : Chemotherapy 3 BEP in case of involved lymph nodes (N+)</td><td colspan="2">1 : Stage II to IV : good prognosis
Chemotherapy – 3 BEP + exeresis of tumoral residue
2 : Stage II to IV : poor prognosis
Chemotherapy / PVeVB
if metastases : Radiotherapy with a palliative aim</td></tr>
<tr><td>non germinal tumours</td><td>For any stage</td><td colspan="2">surgery ± Chemotherapy ± Radiotherapy</td></tr>
</table>

VII. Current results and follow-up

Current results are excellent:

- Cure in more than 95 % of seminoma tumours;
- 5 years survival rate for non-seminoma tumours:
  - Stage I : 90 %
  - Stage III and IV: 70 % if good prognosis, 40 % if poor prognosis

- ***The follow-up:***

During the first two years where recurrences are frequent, we will carry out:

- The dosage of the tumoral markers;
- The chest X-ray;
- The abdominal echography;
- The abdomino-pelvic and chest CT scan;
- The scrotal echography for the follow-up of the contro-lateral remaining testicle by searching for the presence of a secondary cancer at this level and even somewhere else.

This follow-up should be done for a very long term.

VIII. Prospects

- Reduce the frequency of new cancers by alleviating the treatment protocol in stages I (ST and NST);
- Search and systematically treat all cases of cryptorchidy;
- Effectively treat all testicular infections;
- Create a conservative sperm bank for the patients.

Penile cancers

I. Epidemiological specificities

The frequency of penile cancers varies according to countries. This cancer is rare in France and in the Western countries where its incidence ranges from 1 and 1.3 % of male cancers. It is even rarer in African countries particularly in the South of the Sahara; but very frequent in India and in South-East Asia.

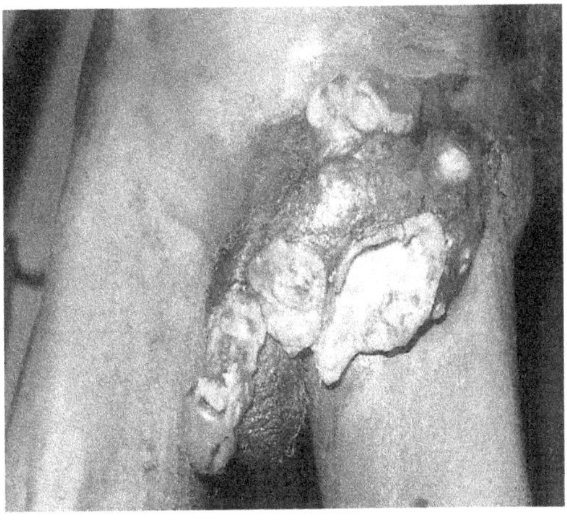

Penile Epidermoïde Carcinoma 60 years old patient

Serology HIV negative, HPV positive

The average age of occurrence is about 60 in the west; 50 in India and even lower (around 40) in Cameroon.

The smegma retention and chronic balanitis appear to be the most favourable factors in Europe than in Africa, where the circumcision from birth is a traditionally respected necessity.

On the contrary, HPV, herpes simplex of type 2, HIV and precancerous dermatological affections, such as the venereal vegetations, huge condyloma acuminata, Bowen and Paget's diseases constitute the favourable factors in developing countries.

II. Diagnostic procedure

The diagnosis time is often very long, one to two years, in African series, in particular.

Indeed, in the frequent absence of any symptoms, even painful ones, it is the tumour itself which most of the time, leads the patient to consult or more rarely phimosis. On the clinical examination, the diagnosis will be strongly suspected in front of an infiltrating, fungating or ulcerating lesion generally located on the glands, close to the balano-preputial furrow; more rarely on the internal side of the prepuce and exceptionally on the sheath of the penis.

The diagnosis is easily confirmed by the histologic study of the biopsy specimen.

The squamous cell carcinoma, most often well differentiated, is the most frequent histologic type; leiomyosarcoma, melanoma and sarcoma except Kaposi are less frequent.

III. Extension assessment

- ***Assessment of the tumour***

The search for signs of local and regional extension of the primary tumour will be easily done by palpation under general anaesthesia. Signs of corpus cavernosum or spongious body and even the urethra infiltration will be noted.

Simultaneous clinical examination, palpation and sometimes fine needle aspiration or biopsy in case of infection of the primary lesion will enable to assess the inguinal lymph nodes extension.

The remote secondary localisations must be systematically searched at the level of bones, the liver and the central nervous system by means of the clinical examination, standard radiography, echography, CT scan and MRI guided as possible by symptomatology.

- ***Assessment of the patient***

The aim is to identify the nature of possible defects, particularly, cardiopulmonary, hepatorenal, immunological and biological; then, to estimate using clinical, para-clinical and biological means, the influence of their effect on the general status of the patient.

IV. Classification and prognostic factors

- *TNM classification*

Stages	Description
Tis	Pre-invasive epithelioma
T0	No clinical sign of primary tumour
T1	Tumours of 2 cm or less in its largest diameter, strictly superficial or exophytic
T2	Tumour of more than 2 cm but less than 5 cm in its highest diameter
T3	Tumour of more than 5 cm in its highest diameter or tumour of any dimension with a deep infiltration including the urethra
T4	Tumour infiltration of surronding organs
Adenopathy	
N0	No palpable Adenopathy
N1	Mobile unilateral Adenopathy
N2	Mobile bilateral Adenopathy
N3	Fixed Adenopathy

- ***Prognostic factors***

The prognosis of penile cancer is related to:

- Primary tumour extension
- Poor histological differentiation
- Young age less than 40
- Poor general status

V. Therapeutic means and methods

- ***The radiotherapy***

Two techniques are often used:

- The external radiotherapy

It is defined as such, because the radioactive source which produces the radiation is placed outside and at a certain distance of the patient. The parameters of irradiation to be determined on the simulator by the specialist are mainly:

-The position of the patient on the treatment machine: the supine position is very often adopted for its simplicity, the patient comfort and especially the reproducibility accuracy all over the treatment time.

- The target volume to be irradiated, generally the entire pelvis including the primary tumour and the pelvic lymph nodes.

- The total dose ranges from 45-50 Gy to 20-30 Gy according to the curative or palliative aim of the treatment.

- The pre-treatment computer-assisted dosimetry whose role in the improvement of the quality and the tolerance of the irradiation is not to be demonstrated any more.

- The interstitial or endo-brachytherapy:

In this technique, the radioactive source is rather directly inserted in the tumour or the tumoral residue in case of partial resection or low- carcinological surgery results.

- ***The surgery***

It is a loco-regional method of treatment, having several techniques:

- The circumcision is necessary in case it is not yet done to fight against infection and to enable an easy examination of the lesion;
- The partial penile amputation with the preservation of a part of corpus cavernosum;
- The total amputation with perineal uretrostomy ;
- Inguino-crural lymph nodes dissection in case of a positive frozen section result;
- The poly-chemotherapy protocol including Bleomycin+ Cisplatin remains unsatisfactory.

VI. Indications and therapeutic protocols

Indications	Protocols
T1T2 ≤4 cm	Endo-brachytherapy
N0	Therapeutic Abstention
N1, N2	Lymph nodes surgery
N-	Abstention
N+	Inguinal radiotheraphy
T2>4 cm T3 T4	Surgery
N3	Lymph nodes surgery
N0	Therapeutic Abstention

VII. Current results/preventive measures and prospects

T1, T2: 5 years Survival Rate: 70 % if N-

The sexual function remains the same as before the treatment. A urethral stricture can be observed in 20 to 40 % of the cases but becomes normal after the dilatation instrumentation.

Possible sequelae in the form of: dyschromy, telangiectasia and superficial sclerosis. The local recurrence period: 5 - 8 years; therefore, it is necessary to plan a long-term follow-up.

T2 > 4 cm T3T4

Unsatisfactory carcinological and conservative treatment results.

3 years SR: 67 % if N +. Nevertheless, frequency of functional and psychological sequelae:

Urethral stricture and impossibility of sexual intercourse.

VIII. Preventive measures

- Circumcision from birth remains the best preventive measure and should be encouraged.
- Treatment of all precancerous lesions should be obligatory as secondary preventive measures.
- Carry research towards the development of more effective radiotherapy and chemotherapy protocols, particularly in advanced stages: big T2 T3 T4 N2 and N3.

PART THREE

HIV/AIDS ASSOCIATED CANCERS

25 years experience in the treatment of HIV/AIDS associated cancers at the Yaounde General Hospital of Cameroon

Introduction

HIV/ AIDS associated cancers are defined as any malignant expansive process of primitive or secondary nature caused in men by a viro-induced immunosuppression.

The current context of this worldwide pandemic and in Cameroon in particular, is marked by a continuous increase in the frequency of HIV infection and associated cancers, mainly due to the non-existence of a preventive or curative vaccine as well as an improvement of life expectancy thanks to the effectiveness of the antiretroviral therapy. Consequently, the fundamental scientific and ethical principle which results from the current level of our knowledge should be expressed by our determination and commitment, for a fully therapeutic medical care with a curative aim already validated by a possible long survival, thanks to antiretroviral treatment. To achieve this goal, we have decided to conduct a retrospective study to assess the protocols and modalities of the treatment applied until now in order to redefine in light of current progress, a more suitable and effective therapeutic approach to HIV/AIDS associated cancers.

To achieve this aim, we did a retrospective and analytical study of 824 patients' medical records, having fulfilled all inclusion criteria, namely: histologically confirmed malignant tumour, HIV positive serology, treatment protocols comprising surgery and/or radiotherapy and/or chemotherapy and systematical antiretroviral treatment.

I. Diagnostic methods of HIV/AIDS associated cancers

1- The first, most available and accessible diagnostic approach of HIV / AIDS associated cancers has been the simultaneous relative long-term follow-up of CD4 cell count kinetic and the frequency of cancers. This kinetic has been in all cases decreasing for CD4 cell count and at the same time increasing for the frequency of cancers; therefore, creating an approximative determinist relation between the onset of cancers and immunodeficient state of the patients.

2- The second approach, certainly the most relevant, would have been to prove by the PCR technique (unfortunately very expensive and therefore, not used systematically), the evidence of the presence of viral genome within cellular genome, particularly of immunocompetent CD4 T-cells.

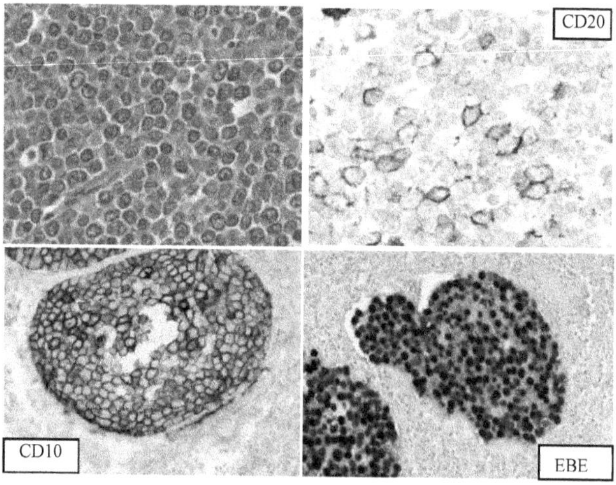

Lymph node lymphoma of bad prognostic: 04 years old child
Histology technics: Hématéine-éosine, immunohistochimie (CD20/10), hybridation *in situ* (EBER)

II. Methods of extension assessment

The approximately complete local, regional and remote extension assessment had been carried out in all cases by clinical, radiological and biological examinations. The pre-therapeutic assessment by clinical, para-clinical and biological means had enabled to evaluate the general health status of patients and to search for defects and opportunistic infections. Finally, the clinical stages of tumours as well as prognostic factor groups (good, poor and intermediary) had been established for every case on the base of the general health status, CD4 cell count, viraemia and the degree of anemia.

III. Therapeutic methods and modalities

At the first step, the curative or palliative aim of the treatment has been decided on the base of prognostic factors.

At the second step, the target volume to be irradiated or operated, the total dose and fractionation modalities, had been adopted and consequently modulated as main parameters of loco-regional methods of treatment by radiotherapy and surgery.

Chemotherapy and hormone therapy, systematic means of treatment were scarcely exclusively used, but most often in association with radiotherapy and surgery according to the protocols adopted in the context of a multidisciplinary approach (Table I).

Table I : Indications and therapeutic protocols

INDICATIONS	THERAPEUTIC PROTOCOLS
Intermediary prognosis Stage T1 T2 Poor general health status Collapse of the immune status CD4 <150 HB < 7 g/dl Massive opportunistic infections Clinical defects+++	**Step 1** No radiotherapy No chemotherapy No surgery Anti-infectious treatment +++ Anti-parasitic treatment blood transfusion ARV prescription+++ **Step 2** Treatment with a curative aim in case of an improvement of clinical and biological parameters **Step 3** Treatment with a palliative aim in case of the persistence of poor prognosis factors
Good prognosis Stage T1 T2 T3 M0 CD4≥200 defects = 0 Opportunistic infections = 0 Good general health status	**Treatment with a curative aim** - Radiotherapy - Surgery - Chemotherapy - ARV prescription+++
Poor prognosis Stage T4 whatever T-N+ M+ CD4<150 Opportunistic infections ±	**Treatment with a palliative aim** - ARV prescription+++ -Anti- infection treatment -Anti-parasitic treatment -other treatments

IV. Statistical analysis of the data and results

- ***Statistical method of analysis***

The survival rate of treated patients was calculated according to the actuarial method and the comparison of this survival rate with that of the patients of the various prognostic groups by the Chi2 test.

- ***Results***

➢ **Oncological description of the patients**

Table II : anatomo-clinical Characteristics of HIV/AIDS associated cancers

<table>
<tr><td colspan="2"></td><th colspan="3">Prognosis factors</th></tr>
<tr><th>Primary tumour</th><th>Histology</th><th>Good prognosis factors</th><th>Intermediary prognosis</th><th>poor prognosis factors</th></tr>
<tr><td>Cervix</td><td>Squamous cells carcinoma</td><td rowspan="6">Stage T1 T2 T3 M0
CD4≥200
defects = 0
opportunistic infections= 0
good general health status</td><td rowspan="6">Stage T1 T2
Poor general health status
Collapse of the immune status CD4 <150
HB < 7 g/dl
Massive opportunistic infections
Clinical defects+++</td><td rowspan="6">Stage T4 whatever T-N+ M+
CD4<150
Opportunistic infections ±</td></tr>
<tr><td>Skin</td><td>Basal cells and spinocellular carcinoma</td></tr>
<tr><td>Lymphoma</td><td>Non Hodgkin's malignant Lymphoma</td></tr>
<tr><td>ENT</td><td>Squamous cells carcinoma</td></tr>
<tr><td>Ano-rectal</td><td>Adenocarcinoma</td></tr>
<tr><td rowspan="2">CNS</td><td rowspan="2">Primary non Hodgkin's lymphoma</td></tr>
<tr><td>N= 248</td><td>N= 138</td><td>N= 438</td></tr>
<tr><th colspan="2">Total</th><th colspan="3">824</th></tr>
</table>

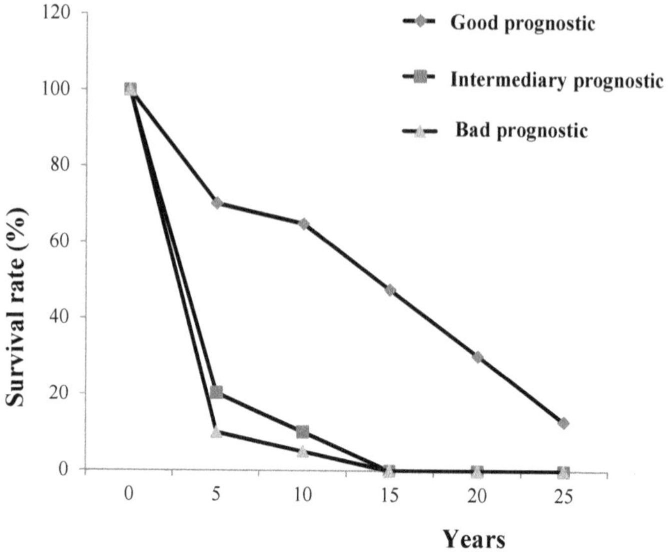

Figure 1 : Variation of the survival rate of patients according to prognostic groups

In summary, the **table II** and **figure 1** show that:

- 438 patients (51,15 %) of the poor prognostic group with very advanced cancer stages T4N+M +, and very poor general health status received a palliative treatment with a survival rate in 5, 10, 15 years of 10 %, 5 % and 0 % respectively.
- 248 patients (30, 1 %) of the good prognostic group, immediately received a radiotherapy with a curative aim, with a survival rate in 5, 10, 15, 20 and 25 years of 70 %,65 %, 48 %, 30 % and 13 % in this order.
- 138 Patients (16, 75 %) of the intermediary prognostic group, received a first line of ARV treatment and other medical care and a second line of treatment was administered with an exclusive

radiotherapy only after an improvement of their general health status.

Their survival rates in 5, 10 and 15 years was 20%, 10 % and 0 % respectively.

Finally, it can be noticed that, the difference of the survival rate is very significant between the various groups of patients with good, intermediary and poor prognosis (p- value <0.001).

Comments:

➤ ***Cytopathogenic and molecular bases***

These bases have already been explained by epidemiological and molecular biology data following the discovery by Montagnier and Gallo of a RNA retrovirus responsible for human immunodeficiency in 1984.

The presence of the viral genome within the genome of immune-competent lymphocytes will be expressed in the form of an insertion, a translocation, an amplification or a mutation of a gene responsible for an induction and cancer transformation.

In this context, the PCR technique, which was not economically accessible to everybody undoubtedly deprives us of an irrefutable proof of the HIV role in the physio pathogenic process of induction of cancers in our serie.

Besides, it has been demonstrated that, the viral genome-cellular genome conflict can lead to the destruction of the immunocompetent cells; therefore, inhibiting the effectiveness of the immune-surveillance system of the internal environment particularly against cancer cells. So, like other authors of literature, the role of HIV was only indirectly suspected following the increase in cancer frequency and parallel reduction of CD4 antibodies.

V. Extension assessment and therapeutic approach

In addition to the usual tumoral parameters of the extension assessment, it is important to note that, the prognostic data of pre-therapeutic assessment such as the level of viraemia, anemia and CD4 cell counts was of vital importance in the therapeutic treatment and have strongly influenced the possibilities of a more or less long survival rate.

They were searched for, with determination, having very well understood that, the quality of a good treatment of which the vital prognosis of the patient depends on, is only possible after their correction which is only possible using ARV drugs and other useful medical treatment support.

Indeed, our results like those of several authors of literature seem, to let us believe (abstraction made on non tumoral prognostic factors), that the survival rate of HIV/AIDS cancers associated patients might be close to those of cancer patients free of HIV [6, 7].

On one hand, the survival rate of these patients in any prognostic group is largely greater (0.9 % in 5 years) than that of the patients of several historic series treated without ARV drugs. On the other hand, it seems to be close to the survival rate of the patients free of HIV.

Conclusion

The aim of this study was to evaluate retrospectively, the treatment protocols and modalities of HIV/AIDS associated cancers at the Yaoundé General Hospital, in order to redefine a more suitable and effective therapeutic approach.

It was a retrospective and analytic study of 824 patients' medical records with an HIV-positive serology, receiving antiretroviral drugs, during the last 25 years for histologically confirmed malignant tumours in the radiotherapy Department of the Yaounde General Hospital.

138 Patients (16, 75 %) of the intermediary prognostic group, received a first line protocol treatment with ARV drugs and supporting medical care.

A second line protocol with an exclusive radiotherapy and/or surgery and/or chemotherapy was done only after a significant improvement of their general health status. Their survival rates in 5 and 10 years was 20% and 10 % respectively.

248 patients (30, 1 %) of the good prognostic group, immediately received a curative radiotherapy, with a survival rate in 5 and 10 years of 70 % and 65 % in this order.

Finally, 438 patients (51,15 %) of the poor prognostic group with very advanced cancer stages T4N+M +, and very poor general health status received only a palliative treatment with a survival rate in 5 and 10 years of 10 % and 5 % in this order.

We still do not have effective means for fighting against cancers in general. The problem is most difficult with those associated with HIV / AIDS. However, only a therapeutic approach privileging a multidisciplinary concertation remains hopefully positive, with the availability of ARV drugs and supporting medical care able to boost the general health status of the patient and the radiotherapy effect, associated or not with surgery and/or chemotherapy, even for poor prognosis cases. Therefore, we should not give up even more discriminate !

PART FOUR

TREATMENT SIDE EFFECTS

Introduction

All cancer treatment methods whether by surgery, radiotherapy or chemotherapy may be at the origin of side effects whose severity can compromise the compliance with the treatment and limit its effectiveness. These effects, not only must be known by the specialists and general practitioners, but also well explained to the patients, the para-medical staffs and NGOs for an early preventive and curative optimal medical, social and psychological care. Therefore, before any treatment, it is advisable to make sure that all the above-mentioned actors understand the fact that, not all patients manifest the same sensitivity to therapeutic complications and also; every patient is individualised by an unpredictable intrinsic sensitivity factor.

According to the international literature data, 10 % of people would present an unusual sensitivity to the radiotherapy favoured by congenital affections involving the DNA defect reparation.

Research programmes are currently being implemented with the hope of developing suitable tests for the pre-therapeutic detection of patients at risks.

I. Specificities of radiotherapy iatrogenic effects

According to the occurrence time, two main lesion groups can be distinguished by their clinical appearances and therapeutic requirements. These two lesions groups are: early or acute, and late or chronic effects.

1- Acute or early Radiotherapy side effects

They occur in the period of time between 0 and 6 months and then, most of the time during the treatment. They are characterised by their organic seat, radiobiological mechanism, clinical aspects and level of severity.

- **cutaneous Complications**

Their frequency varies depending on the energy level of the radiation beam used. It is very low for high energies 4-25 MeV of linear accelerators X-ray; unfortunately not yet accessible in our hospital environments. However, very high for low and average energies, for example 1, 25 MeV of Cobalt 60 gamma-radiation with the almost exclusive use can justify the importance of skin burning in the patients of our series. From tissue friction and maceration, they are frequently visible at the level of folds, particularly the armpit, mammary fissure, inguinal folds and inter-buttock. These skin lesions are mainly observed around the dose of 30 Gy given according to the usual fractionation and staggering of 5x2Gy a week.

Clinically, they first have a sunburn or dry epithelial aspect progressing in an exudative form, then, ulcerated in area to become painful and very uncomfortable. Avoid putting on plastic clothes, no application of any alcoholic or irritant substance; and simply recommend the use of the household soap to have a wash is the main advice to be given to patients being irradiated.

- **mucous membranes Complications**

They are very often embarrassing, in particular at the oral and vaginal level, and may require an interruption of the irradiation resulting in a relatively quick lesion healing.

- **mediastinum Complications**

The main complication is oesophagitis and his pathognomonic symptom is dysphagia, or deglutition pain. The first intention care should be psychological by explaining its mechanism to the patient, and to reassure him/her by confirming that it is a banal and short-lived problem. The nutritional effect will be assessed by the weight control.

➢ Pelvic Complications

Clinically, their presentations are mainly in the form of symptoms of cystitis with dysuria and pollakiuria, then radiation proctitis with tenesmus, derasping and false needs simulating a very acute painful hemorrhoid syndrome. The occurrence of an infectious cystitis is usually well controlled by non-steroidal anti-inflammatory drugs and eventually by urinary antiseptics; and rectitis with, anti-haemorrhoidal drugs and corticosteroid enema.

➢ Painful bone complications

Paradoxically, the well-known inflammatory action of ionising radiations, will rather cause an exacerbation of pains during the first days of treatment, even for radiotherapy of bone metastasis with an analgaesic aim. The analgaesic benefit will only begin 5 to 8 days after the beginning of the irradiation. The patient must be informed and be put concomitantly on oral analgaesic and anti-inflammatory drugs.

➢ Haematological toxicity

Its frequency and seriousness directly depend on the importance of the target volume and therefore on the quantity of haematopoietic marrow effectively irradiated.

Table : Percentage of irradiated bone marrow volume according to the target volume in adults

Target Volumes	Percentage of Bone Marrow
Cervical and dorsal spine	25%
Lumbar spine	25%
Pelvis in particular sacrum	25%
Upper and Lower limbs	25%
Total	100 %

Therefore the control of full blood count should not be systematic, but done according to the importance of the irradiated volume.

It is usually advised to interrupt radiotherapy for the values of white blood cells lower than 2000 and platelet cells lower than 50 000 / mm3 and to carry out a transfusion of units packed cells if the haemoglobin level is lower than 8 mg/dl.

➢ **Complications of the whole-brain irradiation**

The whole-brain irradiation must be carried out under injectable or per os corticosteroid to limit the occurrence of a cerebral oedema that may be the cause of an intracranial hypertension syndrome, particularly disabling.

Alopecia occurs and is irreversible at the total dose of 40 Gy, dose in which sequelae can be seen in the form of psychological and behavioural disorders or seizures. The irradiation side effects are accordingly more severe that it concerns a large volume of the brain and that the prescribed dose is even more important.

2- Radiotherapy late effects

They are defined as side effects or sequelae lesions with a chronic character, which the occurrence time is beyond 6 months.

➢ **Complication of thorax irradiation and lower cervical region**

- Pulmonary fibrosis and post-radiation mediastinum

Constant beyond 20 Gy delivered in classical fractionation of 5x2Gy/week, fibrosis is rarely systematic except when a very large pulmonary volume is irradiated.

Its manifestation is sometime in the form of an exhausted dyspnoea, a chronic cough, fever and asthenia. Most of the time, its expression is purely radiological.

Corticosteroid is a significant support, particularly in the acute clinical stage.

- **Pericarditis**

Pericardial inflammation and even fibrotic is very rarely symptomatic and of good prognosis, except in case of circulatory deficiency with myocardial injury.

- **Radiation plexitis, the big arm and ankylosis of shoulder joint**

Modern techniques of irradiation have been at the base of the disparition of radiation plexitis which involved brachial plexus. However, the big arm and / or ankylosis of shoulder are frequently found in our African series, particularly after radio-surgical treatment of breast cancers including the armpit. The rehabilitation of the joint and lymphatic drainage under analgaesic and anti-inflammatory medication very often lead only to irregular satisfaction results.

- **After-effect or late complications of cerebral irradiation**

At the dose of 40 Gy, after-effects can be expressed in the form of psychological disorders, behavioural problems or seizures. The irradiation is even more harmful that it concerns a large brain volume and that the prescribed dose is also important. It is rare that these late complications occur below 30 Gy whatever the brain volume irradiated according to the classical fractionation of 5x 2 Gy/week.

The quality of radiotherapy certainly depends on the competence of human resources indeed, but also and especially on the performance of technical facilities.

II. Specificities of chemotherapy iatrogenic effects

The direct toxicity, or drug hypersensitivity just like its indirect toxicity, are the two main very dreaded acute or chronic complications of cytotoxic chemotherapy, firstly, because of the non-specific effect of anti-tumoral products on dividing cells ; and secondly, because of infectious, haemorrhagic and immunological consequences of the bone marrow depression.

After more than a decade of research, the targeted therapy has not yet permit to resolve this major handicap for biological and economic reasons, which is very often the cause of a poor treatment compliance, and therefore, of poor results, likely to endanger in short, medium and long terms, the life-prognosis of patients.

- **Complications on mucous membranes, skin and skin appendages**

  - ***Complication on oral mucous membranes***

Mucositis and stomatitis are the most frequent complications met between the 5th and 7th day during chemotherapy.

We remind that two main mechanisms are involved: the direct toxicity of chemotherapy which is the consequence of the non-specific effect of cytotoxic chemotherapy on dividing or mitosis cells and therefore, rapidly renewable. The lesions will be manifested in the form of sore mouth with burns, mucosal erythema, then erosions and ulcerations. The effect on the general state can be important with the installation of a major dysphagia leading to dehydration and undernutrition.

The indirect toxicity of chemotherapy is mainly medullary. It exposes at the risk of superinfection and bleeding oral lesions previously described. This superinfection may be from bacterial or fungal origin, particularly in the form of oral candidiasis.

- The preventive treatment:

Must be initiated before the beginning of chemotherapy using:

- Suitable oral care by a stomatologist;
- A toothbrushing with a simple toothbrush or a cotton swab according to the platelet count;
- Mouthwash at a rate of 3 to 6 times a day with a bicarbonate solution at 14/1000, amphotericin B in suspension.

- The curative treatment:

With an analgaesic aim, by a local application of a viscous xylocaine for instance:

- Antifungal mouthwash;
- Systemic antifungal treatments if necessary;
- Parenteral feeding and rehydration.

  - *Cutaneous complications*

They may occur in the form of serious local complications by extravation during the injections of chemotherapeutics. This incident must be suspected with the beginning of pains at the injection site with burning sensation and the impossibility to obtain a venous return. An inflammatory reaction will secondarily occur and will progress in one week to a necrosis with anatomical dissection and exposed tendons and bones. At this stage, the healing will be long and require several weeks.

The curative treatment will be carried out by the suitable local care and if necessary after surgical resection of necrotic tissue with skin graft.

Many other toxidermia can be observed during chemotherapy:

- Pigmentation disorders which can be presented in the form of a localised or diffuse hyperpigmentation probably after a direct stimulation of melanocytes by the product or its metabolites.
- A photosensitivity can also be observed after some drugs like 5 FU; thus, sun exposure is not recommended.

  - *Skin appendages complications*

- Total or partial alopecia is very frequent. It is fortunately always reversible, despite the significant psychological consequences for some patient. A good information is thus necessary before the beginning of the treatment.
- Disorders can also be observed at the level of nails in the form of a diffuse hyperpigmentation or friable nails with a possible ungula fall.

➢ **Digestive Complications**

Nausea and vomiting constitute the main chemotherapy complications. Clinically we distinguish:

- Acute nausea and vomiting which occur within 24 hours.
- Antiemetisants and Parenteral rehydration very often enable to solve the problem and improve the comfort of the patient.
- Delayed nausea and vomiting begin after the 24th hour. Their duration is variable, from 24 hours to one week. 5HT3, NK1 receptor antagonists and corticosteroids are recommended, in spite of their relative importance in the role of this delayed toxicity.
- Anticipated nausea and vomiting occur within hours or days preceding chemotherapy; the non-productive

vomiting efforts having the same importance as vomiting. They are usually linked to anxiety, young age, female sex, chemotherapy having cisplatin and the increasing number of cycles, especially if they are badly tolerated.

Anxiolytics are recommended in such situations as complementary treatment.

* Diarrhoea can occur as consequences of a direct toxicity of chemotherapy on intestinal mucosa with a short cycle time of cells division. Diarrhoea is reversible in 7 to 10 days after the chemotherapy course of treatment.

* Rehydration, anti-spasmodic and anti-diarrhoeal agents constitute the main components of the curative treatment.

* Neurological toxicity on the autonomic nervous system may be the cause of abdominal pains, with intestinal flow disorders of constipation type able to reach paralytic ileus particularly observed with cisplatin.

➢ **Neurological complications**

The diagnosis of neurological signs during chemotherapy can be asserted only after eliminating other possible aetiologies: bone metastases with secondary neurological complication, brain metastases, a carcinomatous meningitis, the development of a paraneoplastic syndrome.

- Peripheral neuropathies may be manifested by the occurrence of distal paraesthesia at the level of hands and feet, the decrease or abolition of the deep-tendon reflexes, the installation of a para-paresis; more scarcely, an ophtalmoplegia, a diplopia and a peripheral facial paralysis can express cranial nerve injuries.

- Urinary retention, orthostatic hypotension and dysphagia are other signs and symptoms of autonomic neuropathy likely to be worse by the existence of an underlying neuropathy anterior to the initiation of chemotherapy, particularly induced by diabetes, alcoholism and certain neurotoxic drugs.

This toxicity is dose-dependent and can oblige to stop the treatment. The reversibility of these disorders is possible, variable but sometimes after a long period of time.

Therapeutically, the prescription of Rivotril or Tegretol sometimes improves the symptomatology.

- The cerebellar syndrome which is most of the time reversible can occur with high dose of some products like 5 FU. An ataxia, dysarthria, dysmetry, nystagmus or even disorders affecting vigilance are the main signs often observed.

- Encephalopathy is manifested through a mental confusion, hallucinations, anxious agitation, hemiparesis, seizure and coma.

- A cochlear dysfunction and visual disturbances can be observed with the administration of cisplatin and vincristine for instance.

➢ **Cardiovascular complications**

They are usually observed with anthracycline or other cardio-toxic drugs like 5 FU, hence, the importance of a cardiac assessment (ECG, echocardiography) at the beginning of the treatment.

The acute toxicity occurs during the infusion or within the following hours in the form of electrocardiographic modifications, with disorders of auricular or ventricular rhythm, a right axial deviation and a decrease of QRS amplitude. These disorders are often mild and reversible under the treatment.

The late, cumulative toxicity occurs remotely, that is; a few weeks to 5 years after the last injection. It is manifested in the form of a non-obstructive cardiomyopathy with global heart decompensation leading to the patient in 30 to 50% of the cases, despite the beginning of a digital-diuretic treatment.

➢ **Hepatic complications**

Hepato-toxicity can occur in three main forms: toxic hepatitis, the consequence of a cellular toxicity, veino-occlusive disease and more rarely chronic fibrosis.

Biologically, we will observe an increase of transaminase enzymes, mainly associated with steatosis and/or cholestasis. The main diagnostic difficulty remains that of the differential discrimination of secondary localisations, viral and associated drug problems.

A careful supervision assessment of liver function, protein and coagulation assessment are necessary.

➢ **Renal complications**

Uratic toxicity linked to the high production of uric acid and direct renal toxicity of the products used may be the cause of disturbances from a simple moderated increase in serum creatinemia to an acute anuric renal insufficiency requiring the use of haemodialysis.

The preventive measures are essential by maintaining a proper rehydration with forced diuresis; alkalinisation of urine, administration of the acid uric synthesis inhibitors such as Zyloric.

A lyses syndrome due to a brutal and massive cellular destruction in the course of chemotherapy can mainly be observed with big tumoral volume malignant hemopathies (Burkitt lymphoma) and results in the rapid liberation in the blood flow of electrolyte coming from lysed cells. In this context, two complications are to be dreaded: hyperkalaemia that may be fatal and the installation of an acute anuric renal insufficiency due to intra-renal precipitation of calcium phosphate crystals.

Hyperhydration with hyper-diuresis are set as treatment with a preventive aim. Haemodialysis may be necessary in case of vital threat.

- **Other metabolic complications**

In addition to the above-mentioned hyperuricemia, hyperkaliemia and hyperphosphatemia, other metabolic disorders may occur during chemotherapy such as hyponatremia, hypomagnesemia and hypophosphatemia with the administration of vincristine, cyclophosphamide and cisplatin for instance.

All these Ionic deficiencies must be searched and corrected because they are often the etiology of neuromuscular disorders in the form of cramps.

- **Vesical toxicity**

It is described as a dose-dependent and cumulative toxicity which often occurs for high dose of cyclophosphamide and ifosfamide probably through toxic metabolites at the vesical level.

Its clinical signs are mainly hematuric cystitis in the absence of urinary infection and coagulation disorders.

The prevention is based on hyper hydration, hyper-diuresis and the administration of MESNA by intravenous route.

- **Pulmonary complication**

Bleomycine is the responsible agent. Toxicity occurs for cumulative doses of 300 mg.

The clinical symptomatology is late in the form of exertional dyspnoea, dry cough, crépitant groans with infiltrates, less specific to the lung radiography.

The end of treatment is imperative to avoid a diffuse and irreversible interstitial lung fibrosis.

➢ **Medullar toxicity**

This toxicity is the most frequent related to the chemotherapy; it is also among the most premature and results from the destruction of haematopoietic cells during the differentiation process; totipotentes cells constituting the spared medullar reserves.

All the three lineages can be affected. However, the order of appearance of the signs of toxicity will depend on the brevity of the life expectancy of each cells origin. 4 to 5 days for the leukocytes; 8 to 12 days for platelets and 120 days for red blood cells. So, the leuco-neutropenia will constitute the most constant and premature manifestation. The infectious risk is to be feared as soon as polynucleaires is lower than 1000 / mm3. The thrombopenia appears then and comes along with a haemorrhagic risk when the rate of platelets drops to 20 000 / mm3. The affection of the red blood cells with anemia is often late and unstable.

This myelo-toxicity is a dependent dose, non-cumulative and fortunately, very often reversible; but its gravity can vary under influence of certain factors:

- The agent or the chemotherapy protocol used on the precocity or not of the nadir in line with an early medullar toxicity or late sustainable and cumulative with installation of more or less severe reversible disorders require the search for a medullar tumoral cells invasion in the absence of recovery.
- The poor state of the marrow at the initiation of the treatment following the exhaustiveness of medullar

reserves by the multiple chemotherapy and /or previous radiotherapy including an important bone volume.

- The visceral deficiency specially renal and hepatic can come along with a risk of products accumulation or of their toxic metabolites in the body with their increasing toxicity.
- Certain medicinal interactions which can increase the toxicity of anticancerous drugs.
- Obesity which can cause an overestimation of the corporal surface with an overdose; drug distribution in the adipose tissue being low. The reality of the risk of this myelo-toxicity calls for preventive and interventional measures before and during the inter-cure.
- The realisation of a complete hemogramme and the evaluation of the hepatic, renal and cardiac functions
- The hospitalisation for transfusion of globular clots in case of anemia with haemoglobin rate lower than 8 g/dl ; concentrated platelets if obvious bleeding or important thrombopenia with a platelets rate lower than 20 000/mm^3.
- The hospitalisation and broad-spectrum antibiotic treatment in case of febrile neutropenia. An adaptation of doses or a chemotherapy report can be necessary to accelerate the medullar recovery.

The administration of haematopoietic growth factors is very beneficial in case of very aplasiant chemotherapy, in order to decrease the intensity and the duration of the leucopenia, to reduce the infectious risks and to allow in fine the respect of the dose-intensity for better compliance and anti-tumoral effectiveness.

➢ Other haematological manifestations

They are essentially: a haemolysis of immuno allergic or auto-immune mechanism, a particular immunosuppression with some drugs such as the cyclophosphamide and haemostasis disorders, because of the chemical hepato-toxicity followed by the cease in the protein hepatic synthesis, coagulation factors in particular.

➢ Rare iatrogenic effects

- ***Iatrogenic or secondary cancers***

In the West, it represents 0.5 to 3 % of death due to cancer. Their frequency is not well known and should be very low in developing countries, where the survival is very short after a treatment essentially with a palliative aim of the patients seen in about 80 % of the cases in late stages. Indeed, as in the West, an increase in these delayed complications of the chemotherapy should be observed gradually in our hospitable centres with an improvement on curability and survival rates of patients in the early stages, of good prognosis and having benefited from a therapeutic efficiency.

Certain genetic factors seem to predispose the development of the secondary tumours (Transfer of P53; congenital or acquired immunodeficiency).

On the clinical plan, the deadline of the apparition is shorter for the liquid tumours such as the secondary leukaemia, and varies between 2 and 10 years. This deadline is longer for the solid secondary tumours, which are much rarer after the chemotherapy alone and bound essentially to the treatment by radiotherapy.

- ***Gonadic Toxicity***

It is an irreversible major aftereffect which affects the young patients (30-40 years) who would have to accept it unfortunately as some authors will say as reward for their cure; the oligospermia and azoospermia lead to infertility. The cryopreservation of the sperm should be carried out before the chemotherapy, or better more, before the tumoral extension assessment by ionising radiations imaging susceptible to alter the spermatogenesis.

The ovary is more resistant to the chemotherapy; clinically, the ovarian toxicity presents progressively a reversible menstrual irregularity; a reversible amenorrhoea in 50 to 80 % of the cases after 6 to 12 months and finally a definite amenorrhoea with irritability, hot flash and vaginal dryness.

The only preventive measure lies on the choice of medicine and treatment protocols.

The gonadic toxicity of the radiotherapy is an almost endangered complication with the improvement of techniques and modalities of irradiation particularly conformational, guided by the image and with intensity modulation.

It is useful to know that, the exocrine testis is very sensitive to ionising radiations while the leydig cells function is less affected. A dose of 0.08 Gy causes azoospermia and the sterility will be more or less reversible according to the absorbed dose. The dose threshold of sterility irreversibility being 5 Gy.

- ***Sexual Disturbances***

Many causes of sexual disturbances should be known for a better prevention:

- *Iatrogenic physiological Causes*

Sexual impotence is frequent for instance after cysto-prostatectomy for bladder tumours; after total prostatectomy, prostate irradiation or hormone therapy for prostate cancer.

A retrograde ejaculation or an ejaculation may be observed after a lumbar vertebra L2L3L4 lymph nodes dissection.

The pre-therapeutic information and a patient's psychological care after treatment are necessary.

- *Causes due to the specific complications of irradiation*

A dryness and\or a vaginal sclerosis, as well as a cystitis and rectitis are late lesions very often observed after radiotherapy.

The resumption of sexual intercourse with lubricants as early as possible and sufficient oral rehydration with prophylactic antibiotherapy constitute the main measures very often applied.

For haemorrhagic, painful stenosis rectitis, resistant to usual medical care, a left colostomy followed later on by a re-establishment of the continuity of the recto-sigmoid curve could be necessary to accelerate the scarring and the regeneration of the rectal mucosa membrane.

- General health status alteration causes, due to the disease and\or the treatment
- The psycho affective complications of the disease can result from :
    - The uncertainty of the future at the announcement of the diagnosis;
    - The alteration of the body image for example after mastectomy, hysterectomy, colostomy or some side effects of the chemotherapy (alopecia, nausea, vomiting) ;
    - Anxiety at the end of the treatment due to the fear of a recurrence.

BIBLIOGRAPHY

1. ACT_UP-PARIS. (2005). L'Epidémiologie à l'infection à VIH/SIDA dans le monde. www.actuparis.org.

2. ANGWAFO F., YOMI J., MBAKOP A. (1994). Is cancer of the prostate rare in tropical (black) Africa ? Case series from the Centre Hospitalier et Universitaire and the Hospital General de Yaoundé from 1986 to 1990. *Bulletin cancer/radiothérapie*, 81 : 155-159.

3. GARRAIT V, MOLINA J. (2000). Infection par VIH : Epidémiologie, dépistage, prévention, principales anomalies immunologiques, marqueurs pronostiques, biologiques, Classifications (stades évolutifs). *La Revue du praticien,* 50 : 1003-6.

4. KENFANG N., YOMI J., KASIA J.M. et.al. (2011). Breast cancer profile in a group of patients followed up at the radiation therapy unit of Yaounde General Hospital, Cameroon. *Obstetrics and gynecology international*, article ID143506.

5. LARTIGAU E. (2009). *Radiothérapie Oncologique : Concepts, techniques et applications cliniques*, John Libbey Eurotext.

6. LEWDEN C, SALMON D, MORLAT P, BEVILACQUA S. (2004). Causes de décès des personnes infectées par le VIH en 2000 : persistance du SIDA, rôle émergent des cancers et des hépatites. *Bulletin Epidémiologique*.

7. MAZERON J-J., MAUGIS A., BARRET C., MORNEX F. (2005). *Techniques d'irradiation des cancers : la radiothérapie conformationnelle*. Maloine.

8. MBOPI FX, VOUNDI E, KALLA GC, EMAH I, ANGWAFO F, MUNA W. (2014). Facteurs influençant l'initiation du traitement antirétroviral des personnes vivant avec le VIH dans les centres de traitement agréés de Bamenda et de Bertoua au Cameroun (epidemiological investigation report 2 : 1-7).

9. National Cancer Institute. (2010). *AIDS-Related Lymphoma Treatment Professional Version. Bethesda*.

10. Organisation Mondiale de la Santé (OMS). (2010). *Traitement antirétroviral de l'infection à VIH chez l'adulte et chez l'adolescent : recommandations pour une approche de santé publique*. Genève.

11. Organisation Mondiale de la Santé (OMS). (2013). *Le Point 2013 de l'OMS sur le traitement de l'infection à VIH dans le monde : Résultats, impact et opportunités*.

12. PREAU M, MARCELIN, CARRIERI MP. (2007). Health related quality of life in french people living with HIV in 2003 (results from the national ANRS-EN12-VESPA study 21(1): 19-27).

13. RAKOWCZ-SZULCZYNSKA E., MCINTOSH DG., PERRY MJ. (1995). Mechanisms of cancer growth promotion by HIV-I neutralizing antibodies. *The Cancer journal*.

14. TAMBOURING P. (1991). *Biologie des cancers*, Marketing/Eclipses.

15. TRIBONNIERE X, PUGLIESE P, CABIE A, CUZIN L, BILLAUD E, POIZOT-Martin I et al. (2007). Caractéristiques démographiques, cliniques, immunovirologiques et thérapeutiques de 8714 patients infectés par le VIH de la cohorte NADIS en 2006.

16. TUBIANA M., DUTREX J., WAMBERSIE A. (1986). *Radiobiologie*, Hermann.

17. VINCENT T., DEVITA JR., HELLEMAN S., ROSENBERG. (2001). *Cancer : principles and practices of oncology*, 6th ed., Lippincott Williams & Wilkins.

18. YOMI J. (1999). Difficultés de l'approche diagnostique et thérapeutique des cancers du testicule dans un pays en développement : à propos d'un cas chez un enfant camerounais de 8 ans. *Cahiers santé*, 9 :329-331.

19. YOMI J. (2017). After nearly thirty years of radiation oncology in Cameroon, regression or progress ! *Bulletin cancer/radiothérapie*, 21 : 398-399.

20. YOMI J., ANGWAFO III, FOUDA A. et.al. (1992). La radiothérapie, médicament essentiel de la douleur cancéreuse dans les pays en développement. *Bulletin cancer/radiothérapie*, 79 :279-283.

21. YOMI J., ATENGUENA E., TABOLA L. (2014). Traitement de la douleur cancéreuse à l'Hôpital Général de Yaoundé. *Health science disease*, 15(2).

22. YOMI J., GONSU FJ. (1995). Causes sociales, économiques et éducationnelles du diagnostic et du traitement tardif des cancers au Cameroun. *Bulletin cancer*, 82 :724-727.

23. YOMI J., MINLO J., SAMBA NGAMO O., PAGBE JJ. (2014). Traitement des cancers associés au VIH/SIDA. *Cancérologie Clinique en Afrique*, 1 : 40-43.

24. YOMI J., MONKAM G., TAGNI D., DOH A. (1996). Prise en charge thérapeutique des cancers du col utérin à Yaoundé à propos d'une série de 111 malades. *Médecine tropicale*, 56 : 159-162.

25. ZOUNG-KANYI, NJE T., ABENA P. (2014). Guide national de prise en charge des personnes avec le VIH/SIDA-Cameroun (epidemiological investigation report).

CONTENTS

LITTÉRATURE GÉNÉRALE, MÉDECINE, SANTÉ, PSYCHIATRIE AUX ÉDITIONS L'HARMATTAN

Dernières parutions

HISTOIRE D'OS

Mémoires d'un chirurgien orthopédiste (1959/2017)

Gérard Alexandre

Ces brèves indépendantes les unes des autres, l'auteur retracent de l'intérieur avec un humour rabelaisien une série de situations et de portraits d'un monde mal connu. Par touches successives, le lecteur découvrira la vie agitée d'un interne, des portraits de chirurgiens, de patrons et de mandarins. Il verra le regard que porte le professionnel sur l'évolution de son métier, sur ses patients, les cas difficiles qu'il doit traiter, les situations cocasses qu'il rencontre, les milieux divers où il évolue. C'est le quotidien d'un métier riche en émotions de tous genres que le lecteur est invité à partager.

(Coll. Médecine à travers les siècles, 282 p., 28 euros)

ISBN : 978-2-343-15617-0, EAN EBOOK : 9782140098871

ÉLÉMENTS D'HYGIÈNE ET ASSAINISSEMENT DU MILIEU APPROFONDIS

Prévention et santé publique tropicale

Berry Kapya Lubamba

L'hygiène et l'assainissement du milieu s'inscrivent dans le cadre général de santé publique en amont des problèmes sanitaires et, comme le cas de la République Démocratique du Congo le démontre, il est important de les considérer comme des éléments de prévention au même titre que les vaccinations ou la protection maternelle et infantile.

(144 p., 23 euros)

ISBN : 978-2-336-31208-8, EAN EBOOK : 9782140054211

LE FLEUVE DE MA MÉMOIRE

Itinéraire d'un médecin d'Afrique

Emmanuel Eben-Moussi

Dans Le fleuve de ma mémoire, Itinéraire d'un médecin d'Afrique, Emmanuel Eben-Moussi convoque le passé et le présent à travers souvenirs et anecdotes. L'auteur tente de décrypter les nouveaux enjeux de terrain, et propose de nouvelles approches de formation et éducation médicales. Il décrit des itinéraires de vie, dans un monde à identités multiples, mais aussi fracturé face à l'instabilité.

(Coll. Écrire l'Afrique, 230 p., 22 euros)

ISBN : 978-2-343-12960-0, EAN EBOOK : 9782140050930

L'EXPÉRIENCE D'UN MÉDECIN DE SANTÉ PUBLIQUE AU BURKINA FASO

Brahima Michel Sombie

Cet ouvrage est le témoignage d'un acteur important du développement du système de santé du Burkina Faso.

(Coll. Harmattan Sénégal, 242 p., 24,5 euros)

ISBN : 978-2-343-12914-3, EAN EBOOK : 9782140049095

Structures éditoriales du groupe L'Harmattan

L'Harmattan Italie
Via degli Artisti, 15
10124 Torino
harmattan.italia@gmail.com

L'Harmattan Hongrie
Kossuth l. u. 14-16.
1053 Budapest
harmattan@harmattan.hu

L'Harmattan Sénégal
10 VDN en face Mermoz
BP 45034 Dakar-Fann
senharmattan@gmail.com

L'Harmattan Cameroun
TSINGA/FECAFOOT
BP 11486 Yaoundé
inkoukam@gmail.com

L'Harmattan Burkina Faso
Achille Somé – tengnule@hotmail.fr

L'Harmattan Guinée
Almamya, rue KA 028 OKB Agency
BP 3470 Conakry
harmattanguinee@yahoo.fr

L'Harmattan RDC
185, avenue Nyangwe
Commune de Lingwala – Kinshasa
matangilamusadila@yahoo.fr

L'Harmattan Congo
67, boulevard Denis-Sassou-N'Guesso
BP 2874 Brazzaville
harmattan.congo@yahoo.fr

L'Harmattan Mali
Sirakoro-Meguetana V31
Bamako
syllaka@yahoo.fr

L'Harmattan Togo
Djidjole – Lomé
Maison Amela
face EPP BATOME
ddamela@aol.com

L'Harmattan Côte d'Ivoire
Résidence Karl – Cité des Arts
Abidjan-Cocody
03 BP 1588 Abidjan
espace_harmattan.ci@hotmail.fr

L'Harmattan Algérie
22, rue Moulay-Mohamed
31000 Oran
info2@harmattan-algerie.com

L'Harmattan Maroc
5, rue Ferrane-Kouicha, Talaâ-Elkbira
Chrableyine, Fès-Médine
30000 Fès
harmattan.maroc@gmail.com

Nos librairies en France

Librairie internationale
16, rue des Écoles – 75005 Paris
librairie.internationale@harmattan.fr
01 40 46 79 11
www.librairieharmattan.com

Librairie l'Espace Harmattan
21 bis, rue des Écoles – 75005 Paris
librairie.espace@harmattan.fr
01 43 29 49 42

Lib. sciences humaines & histoire
21, rue des Écoles – 75005 Paris
librairie.sh@harmattan.fr
01 46 34 13 71
www.librairieharmattansh.com

Lib. Méditerranée & Moyen-Orient
7, rue des Carmes – 75005 Paris
librairie.mediterranee@harmattan.fr
01 43 29 71 15

Librairie Le Lucernaire
53, rue Notre-Dame-des-Champs – 75006 Paris
librairie@lucernaire.fr
01 42 22 67 13

www.ingramcontent.com/pod-product-compliance
Lightning Source LLC
Chambersburg PA
CBHW071344230926
51846CB00002B/438